THE PURSUIT OF FAMILY

HOW ONE COUPLE, TWO JUDGES, AND THREE WOMBS MADE A FAMILY OF SIX

JULIE AGUAS

Introduction

Family. It seems like a simple enough pursuit. We've all heard the lyric, "First comes love, then comes marriage..." We know what comes next. It's only natural. Dogs, rats, even cockroaches seamlessly accomplish this feat on a daily basis. According to science, to be living, a thing must be capable of growth, reproduction and metabolism. I've got growth and metabolism down cold. It's the reproduction part that boxes me out of the club of the living. So I am left to exist with the in-between things, like fire, in the 2/3 living category.

I am not the only one who fails to meet the basic criteria for life. But it sure can feel like I am. That is because we in-between people tend to cover up our gaping holes in shame. We look and act like everyone else, so many would never guess that we are actually 1/3 missing. Close friends do not know our stories. They might know some of the facts. They might guess at some of the details. But from their vantage point - a very stiff-arm's length from us - how can they truly know? It is no wonder that we are an isolated and misunderstood group. It is no wonder that people don't know how to respond to us.

I spent seven long years stretching and contorting myself to will that missing 1/3 into existence. I thought that if I pushed hard enough, I could expand myself to form to the boundaries of the mold and join with my cockroach brothers and sisters in the world of the living. But eventually I learned that the only things I truly had the power to change were my own definitions. So I set about redefining for myself the meaning of life, of family, of God. It was only then that I could even begin to accomplish my mission.

I don't want to be alone anymore. I want to tell you my story as I experienced it. I want you to see my holes and what I have built around them. If you have holes too, then you will know that you are not alone. My story begins like many others - with a naïve young girl who believes that the world is fair…

Chapter 1
In Good Times

As we rounded the corner, the thunderous crackle and explosion of colors ceremoniously lit the way to what would be our home together as a married couple. It was as if the fates had secretly convened during our weekend together in San Francisco to decide upon the ultimate welcome-home display for a newly-engaged couple.

"Fireworks!" James and I gazed at the sky through a layer of emerging tears. "God must really approve of us!"

Of course, it *was* Labor Day weekend, and the local amusement park traditionally closed out the occasion with a fireworks extravaganza. But why split hairs - it was so much more romantic to see it as a private show meant only for us. And why not see it that way? God probably didn't arrange the show itself, but couldn't He have arranged the timing of our journey home so as to land us at that perfect spot, right at that perfect moment? Why not?

Yes, our life was going to be the stuff of legends. Not the legends that contained strife and tragedy, because that part of the journey was over. I had been through the many lonely nights of looking up to the heavens and asking why every person on earth had a soul-mate except for me. I had even reached the ripe old age of 24 without ever once falling in love (with the obvious exception of Antonio Sabato Jr.). I certainly had paid my dues of suffering, and it was time to reap some rewards. Looking back on it all, I could see that the suffering was well worth it because it had built my character, transforming me into the mature, self-actualized adult I beheld in the mirror.

Prior to my recent enlightenment, I had looked at things much differently. I had once seen my failure to survive life as a high school math teacher as a soul-crushing disaster. But now I could see that peeking out just behind the dark veil of perceived tragedy was a brilliant bouquet of unexpected blessings. My necessary suffering had led me to a new, exciting career as a software engineer. And of course most importantly, it led me to meet James, the love of my life.

The first time I caught sight of James, I was brand new at work. I was fumbling through some software tests, feeling a little lost in the new lingo and a little bored from the long stretches of sitting. The coffee I had been sipping was no longer having any effect due to the tolerance built up after days of chugging to stay awake. I looked up as he entered the room, and my body had a jolt of caffeine-equivalence. He was stunningly good looking, with a broad, muscular build. His eyes transmitted a wave of sincerity, with a little flicker of mischief. As he spoke to a coworker, I was awed by his fluency and ease with the technical words that I was still struggling to learn.

The coworker glanced over at me.

"Oh hey, Julie, I'd like you to meet James Aguas. James, this is our new hire, Julie Trayer."

I quickly assessed my appearance. Was my mouth gaping open? Were my eyes watering from staring at the computer screen? I stood up and shook James' hand, and it felt strong and warm in my own. Things were looking a lot less boring at work!

My crush on James grew exponentially with each interaction. We had gotten to know each other gradually over lunches with coworkers, break-time ping pong matches, and email exchanges here and there. James' emails were so cute and clever that I would find myself spending 20 minutes to craft a two-sentence response to him. James was constantly sending me into embarrassing fits of giggling. In his presence, I felt like a giddy teenager. As I got to know him, I also learned that we shared common values. Like me, he was a practicing Catholic who found a moral compass within his own heart rather than in doctrine. He spoke lovingly of his mother and four siblings and would drop whatever he was doing any time they needed his help. Visits to the office from his adorable two year old niece gave me a sneak peek into his natural paternal tenderness. After so many years of searching, I had found a man who not only aced every bullet point of my stringent marriage-material checklist, but also transformed my list-driven brain into a heap of blushing, quivering mush.

Of course there were some minor hurdles to overcome. For one thing, James had a girlfriend. Finding that out was a major disappointment. But I bided my time, and within a couple of months, James sadly announced their break-up. I gave proper condolences, and silently did an inner cartwheel-back handspring (sticking the landing brilliantly, by the way). At that point, I gave myself the go-ahead to actively pursue him. I invited him to join my church choir, and to my surprise, he agreed. A couple of choir practices were enough to get us to admit our feelings for one another and to share our first trembling, awkward kiss. From that moment on, I knew that I would be married to James Aguas. Of course, it took him nearly three years to come to the same conclusion and propose to me. But I was patient (don't ask him, he probably wouldn't vouch for me on that one), and my moment arrived when James Aguas, with the Bay Bridge as his back-drop and the gentle waves lapping in approval, dropped to one knee and asked me to be his wife.

In February, James and I attended our compulsory Catholic engagement classes, which began with us filling out separate surveys. The questions attempted to assess our level of discussion and agreement on major life issues. I was thrilled when I found out the class started with this test. Bump us straight up to the head of the class – we were going to ace this one! Our countless long talks must have at least scratched the surface of every major topic that existed. When the priest handed back our tests, I eagerly read our results. Well, it wasn't quite a perfect paper. There was one topic which we had not discussed and were not yet in sync on. The question was, "have you discussed what you would do if one or both of you were unable to produce children." All of the couples were sent to various points around the room to discuss the test results.

"So what about that fertility question?" I said to James. "What would you want to do if one of us couldn't produce a child?"

James furrowed his brow, "Well, I hate to even think about that, but if we couldn't produce a child, then I would still want a family, so I would definitely want to adopt."

I considered what he had said. To be honest, the thought had never occurred to me that having a family with James would be anything but simple. James and I were both healthy, and no one in our family suffered from fertility problems.

I already had some experience with adoption because I was raising a little girl who was not biologically my own. Marsha was a seriously-neglected child of a neighbor. Knowing the instability of her family, I had initially entered her life to check on her and make sure that her needs were being met. I ended up falling in love with her, and she came to live with me full time at 2 ½ years old. Due to all of the neglect and trauma that she had endured, Marsha had been an extremely difficult toddler. She had been violent and erratic, at one point averaging 20 tantrums per day. But underneath, her true self always shone through stronger than the damaged parts. As the years whittled off more of the trauma, she gradually evened out. At this point it would not be exaggerating to say that she was the most delightful 11-year old I'd ever met. Marsha was generous with hugs and accepting of all people. She had an endearing innocence which rendered her literally incapable of lying or comprehending why anyone would. I knew that the love I felt for her was as strong as the love that I could feel for a biological child, so I quickly concluded that if God forbid, things didn't work out biologically, adoption would be the natural next step.

"Yes, I agree with that," I responded to James. And with that, we aced Catholic Marriage 101.

Our eight month engagement flew by, and we found ourselves at the altar on April 26, 2003. That year it had rained the entire month of April, very uncharacteristic of our sunny pocket of California. But on April 26, the sun shone brightly, and the rain took a one day leave of absence just for us. Our wedding was beyond perfect. Father Gilbert performed the ceremony. He was new to the parish, but we had gotten to know him well over the course of our engagement. Ours was the first wedding that he had ever presided over. He did a beautiful job, with the occasional misspeak - "Now that you have declared your descent...I mean consent!" or forgotten cue – he forgot to say "You may now kiss the bride." But every little mishap just added to the charm of the ceremony. The same church choir which had provided my initial excuse to get to know James was now emitting spirited tones that enveloped the room with the embrace of an old friend. When it came time to say our vows, I had to go first. I was petrified that I would forget my lines or start bawling. Amazingly, I made it through, just choking up on the very last phrase, "All the days of my life." James' turn came next, and he strongly burst out with the first couple of lines. Then he started the phrase, "In good times..." He paused for an instant, "And in bad." Now his voice was cracking. "In sickness...and." At this point, he was unable to continue. I started hearing sniffling in the crowd behind me, and it seemed inevitable that we were going to have the whole room in tears. I knew if I started crying, I'd never stop, so I bit my lip and held on. James turned to the congregation and smiled, making a "timeout" gesture with his hands. The entire room burst out laughing, breaking through the tension of the moment. At this point, he pulled himself together and completed his vows like a champion.

James was not simply reciting vows. With each word, he was acknowledging the meaning and gravity of what he was saying. We would be together forever, supporting one another through everything. To us at this blissful moment, "bad times" was an abstract concept of the inevitable tragedies of life, like losing an aged loved one or a family pet. Neither

James nor I had any idea of how soon we would be forced to live up to those vows.

    I did not cry a single tear on my wedding day despite the fact that they were flowing in torrential downpour around me. And I am a natural crybaby, known to well up over a Hallmark card, so it took a dam the size of the Great Wall of China to hold those tears back. James paid for it dearly the next day when the dam gave way, and I sobbed straight through a flight to Florida followed by a flight to St. Thomas. He kept asking me, "Are you OK?" to which I responded amid sniffles and snorts, "I'm just so happy!" We averted our eyes from the stares of the flight attendants who must have been concocting their own theories about my frazzled state. By the time we reached St. Thomas, James' "beautiful" bride was a puffy-eyed, blotchy-faced mess, appearing to be on her way to a funeral!

    But our honeymoon was anything but funeral-like. We hiked, scuba dived, strolled, ate, and enjoyed life together. We talked about our future, how perfect our children would be. We couldn't wait to start a family – heck, we had the names of our babies picked out long before we were even married! A boy would be called Isaac, and our little girl would be Natalie. We didn't know exactly what they would be like, but we knew one thing for sure - the two of us morphed into a child would be far superior to the separate individuals. Our trip to purchase glasses a few months back had demonstrated that fact. James, having a large head and a wide face, had to try on every pair of men's glasses in the entire store before finding a single pair that fit his face. I also had to sample the complete inventory of women's glasses due to my face being too narrow. Our children, however, would have the perfect dimensions, such that each pair they tried on would look just as cute as the next. Where I lacked, James excelled, and vice versa. And there were a few genetic contributions that we both could bring to the table. We shared a deep love of music and enjoyed singing and playing instruments. One of our favorite activities was jamming together, me on the piano, and James on the drums. We imagined our little brood of Von Trapps, each an expert in a particular instrument – the whole family making beautiful music together.

Returning from paradise, James and I were energized and ready to experience real married life. We were greeted by Marsha, who was now referring to James as "Dad." And I of course exploited every opportunity to refer to myself as "Mrs. Aguas." Life for the newly-born Aguas family settled into a happy routine.

Within a month of the wedding, I began laying the groundwork for the expansion of our family. I started dropping subtle hints here and there that I wanted to try to get pregnant (if you consider a stadium sized jumbo-tron flashing, "Let's make a baby!!!" subtle). At the advanced age of 27, I was surely teetering on the edge of my peak fertility years and was eager to get started before it was too late. James also wanted to get started soon, but he figured we should at least wait a few months. A few months it was – by the beginning of July, I had taken my last birth control pill.

I come from a long line of women who got pregnant on their very first month of trying. If they set their minds to it, my mother, grandmother and aunt could probably get pregnant without a man. I could only assume that I would be the same. To add to my advantage, I had always been able to feel that distinctive pinch in the side that meant that I was ovulating. There would be no guesswork involved.

By the end of that first month of trying, I was already speculating on the state of our potential embryo, feeling intently for a sign of his or her existence. Never was urination as thrilling as when I baptized my first pregnancy test stick. James and I sat side by side, watching for that second blue line to surface. The test kit said that it would take two to three minutes, so we quietly stared, hearts pounding, giddy with anticipation. At last, two minutes passed, then three, then four. But no matter how we squinted or held it up in better light, the lonely first line was all that would deign to appear. The honeymoon was officially over.

Chapter 2
The Elusive Blue Line

Months passed, and James and I were still on the hunt for the elusive blue line. Panic began to set in. I knew very little about how fertility treatments worked, but I had heard that couples are normally required to try for a full year before specialists will even let them in the door to start testing and treating infertility. I could never wait a whole year – totally unacceptable! So I poured my efforts into learning about what we could do to increase our chances each month. I modified my diet, gave up caffeine, gobbled down as many vitamins as I could, took my basal temperature every morning, and hung practically upside-down after sex. James and I even got private lessons from a Natural Family Planning expert. Not the sort of thing that Grandma ever did!

I began to observe a curious phenomenon that I have since coined the Great Plague of Belly Swelling. There was clearly something in the air or the water supply that was causing uncanny fertility in the overall population. And for some excruciatingly mysterious reason, I was the only one with complete immunity to it. Every person I knew was calling me with a stirring announcement of the fruits of their fertility. A coworker proclaimed that triplets were on the way. Ten, twenty times a day, I would encounter strangers with that unmistakable glow and expanding waist-line. Even movie stars seemed to be cranking out the babies at an uncommonly high rate. When I visited my general practitioner to get checked out for any potential issues, she waddled in the door – at least seven months along! What was going on? What did they know that I didn't?

Thanksgiving came and went. Christmas came and went. My brother-in-law had been planning a March wedding in the Philippines, which I had assumed that I wouldn't be able to attend due to a pregnancy. As March approached, it was clear that the chances of conceiving before the trip were dwindling away. So I booked my flight and joined the rest of the family.

My opportunity to visit to the Philippines was the one silver lining of our fertility failures. In James' home province of Pampanga, I soaked up the people and places that had formed the first ten years of his life. Marsha got to experience one of James' early household chores as she pumped water by hand from the same pump that he had used as a child. We visited his elementary school in Bacolor that had been destroyed by the eruption of Mt. Pinatubo. A nearby church called San Guillermo had been half buried in volcanic ash, yet the heart-strong congregation had simply built a new floor and continued their worship with lower windows and ceiling. At the church, we purchased a figurine of a man and woman with a tiny baby nestled in their arms. The piece was made of the very volcanic ashes that had destroyed so much. As I stroked its smooth lines, I set my mind on transforming the ashes which had invaded my life into beautiful works of art. My new revelation reigned in my racing thoughts. I pondered the fact that James and I had grown up so far apart and with vastly different circumstances. What a powerful stroke of fate must have carefully directed each of our lives such that we would eventually meet one another. This force would continue to take care of us, and in the end, everything would work out. We just had to do our best with the hand we were being dealt, and at some point (of course hopefully a point within the next few months), things would work out.

Marsha and I returned home from the Philippines a week before James so that Marsha could return to school. Since this was the first time that James and I had been apart since we'd been married, we lingered on the phone each night lamenting how much we missed one another. Eventually, I would start falling asleep mid-sentence, signaling that it was time to hang up. At work, the days were dragging as I struggled against both jet-lag and sleep deprivation.

James returned home a couple of days before my period was due, and I started feeling the familiar cramping that signaled yet another failure. It had been nine months since we had started trying, so soon we would qualify for a fertility evaluation. Each time the panic started creeping in, I would gaze at the "Family of Ashes" we had bought in the Philippines, and I would try to visualize our adversity being transformed. My 28th birthday arrived, yet another reminder of the steadily closing window that I so desperately wanted to slip through.

On the morning of March 21, I woke abruptly at 3:00 am. Figuring this unwanted reveille was a relapse of jet-lag, I nestled my head into the pillow and attempted to go back to sleep. But something was nagging at me in a corner of my drowsy mind. Rubbing my eyes, I tried to remember what day it was. My heart caught on a couple of seconds before my brain and started pounding audibly. My period was two days late!

I scrambled out of bed. Stabilizing myself, I made my way to the bathroom. Gently closing the door, I flicked on the light, stunning my eyes with the sudden brightness. I still had one home pregnancy test left from last month. Squinting, I whipped it out of the drawer and pulled out the test stick, which was sealed in heavy plastic. My hands were in an exasperatingly sleepy state, unable to muster enough grip to rip open the plastic. Focusing all of my energy toward my hands, like a jedi summoning a light saber from across the room, I willed them to grasp. The plastic began to give way. I pulled out the stick and held it firmly in a steady stream of urine. Glancing at my watch, I braced myself for the two-minute wait. Suddenly, about 30 seconds in, I spotted a hint of a shadow against the white background of the test window. Gradually the shadow darkened and formed as an unmistakable second blue line. My breathing skipped and stuttered, and tears pooled in my eyes. The agonizing wait was finally over! I swung open the door and hurled myself into the bed, startling James into an upright position.

"What's wrong! What's going on!" he gasped.

"Sweetie, it's positive! It's positive!!"

Even though I hadn't told him what the heck was positive, he immediately knew. We fell into each other's arms, crying and laughing at the same time.

"It's perfect," James chuckled, "Made in the Philippines."

By the time the sun had peeked over the horizon that morning, James and I had called at least five family members, their drowsy hellos followed by screams of elation. When Marsha woke up, we sat her down and told her of her impending sibling.

Now Marsha had been begging me for a sibling ever since she was a tiny girl. She actually had six biological siblings who were scattered with various family members, but she had desperately wanted a sibling to live with her. Around the age of six, she began enlisting strangers to help her achieve her goal.

"Are you married?" she once asked a middle aged man she met at a company party. She was amused by the man, whose behavior had been growing increasingly raucous in direct proportion with the alcohol in his bloodstream.

"No," the man responded. Technically he wasn't married, although he was attending the party with a girlfriend and two teenaged children from his previous marriage.

"Well, then would you like to marry my mommy?" she proposed, head cocked, arms folded across her chest, "She is a spinster."

The man chuckled, and opened his mouth to respond when I abruptly cut him off. "Sorry about that," I mumbled as I ushered Marsha away from the *gentleman*.

Luckily when Marsha met James, she found him to be every bit as desirable as Middle-Aged Funny Man. Not long after their first meeting, Marsha ever so casually mentioned to James that she would like him to be her daddy.

By the time James and I walked down the aisle, Marsha's desire for a daddy had not diminished, but she had gradually come to the conclusion that a new sibling was not in her best interest. Quite accustomed to being the only child and only grandchild on my side of the family, she was not eager to give up her comfy position as the cutest thing around. Plus, she figured quite accurately, that a newborn baby wouldn't make an ideal playmate for a 12 year old. At one point, she asked me to consider adopting a 12 year old instead of having a baby with James.

But being the gracious child that she is, Marsha forced a smile when we told her about the baby. We took her out for a special breakfast to celebrate. As I sipped hot cocoa with my two favorite people in the world, I was filled with certainty that her heart would open to our child once she got used to the idea.

When the weekend ended, we returned to work. Even though we were bursting with our news, we only told a couple of coworkers. But like any good piece of gossip, the word of our pregnancy quickly spread. Pretty soon, virtual strangers were passing me in the hallways of our office saying, "Congratulations!" I didn't mind, figuring the more people praying for our baby, the better.

Chapter 3
The Noble Rite

Some women wish that there was a simple way to achieve the end product of a biological baby without experiencing nine months of pregnancy – the weight gain, the queasy stomach, the mind-altering hormonal surges, the unbearable pain of childbirth. Not me! I was looking forward to every facet of the experience. Since I had been a small child, I had revered the state of pregnancy and eagerly anticipated the glorious transformation of my body. What a miracle it would be to bond with this tiny being as it gradually made its presence known. Even if pain were involved, it was a necessary part of this noble rite of passage. I felt sorry for men that they were deprived of the experience.

By my fifth week of pregnancy, the smile on my face was indelible. I could swear that my belly was poking out ever so slightly. I was noticing increased fatigue during the day, which I saw as a wonderful excuse to take things easy. All was right with the world as I read my first of many pregnancy books, lounging on a lawn chair under the blossoming crabapple tree, treating my growing baby to the gentle warmth of the spring sun.

One Sunday morning, as I showered, I started to sense something wasn't quite right. I quickly finished my shower and dried off. My face felt cold and clammy. My steps were unsteady. Suddenly I felt a jarring spasm in my abdomen. I rushed for the toilet and the contents of my stomach willfully made their way to the local water-treatment plant. Feeling instantly better, I washed out my mouth and raced to the bedroom.

"Sweetie, Sweetie!" I shouted, again startling my long-suffering husband out of a peaceful sleep.

"What! Is everything alright?" James' eyes darted about the room, scanning for the source of the commotion.

"I just had my first bout of morning sickness!" I proudly proclaimed.

"Yes Sweetheart." James drowsily responded. "Congratulations, I think," he mumbled as he drifted back to sleep.

I must admit however that my enthusiasm for morning sickness waned very quickly over the next few weeks. My nausea would not accept the rigid confines of morning, and generously spread itself through the entire day. It didn't come in waves like I had expected, but was there constantly, hovering over me. Ordinarily a lover of all things food, I could no longer stand the sight, or especially the smell of anything edible. I spent each endless work day continuously prying my head off my desk, trying to muster up some semblance of productivity. Evenings were spent scouring the internet for morning sickness remedies. The articles I read held some promise of feeling human again by the end of the first trimester, though some accounts told of the unrelenting ailment lasting the entire nine months! Over the course of my life, I had suffered the occasional stomach flu, which had never lasted longer than a couple of days. I had always ridden it out in bed, my awareness of the suffering fluctuating as I drifted in and out of sleep. I had never even considered getting up and going to work in such a state! How did women do it?

Trudging through my work days with or without my stomach's cooperation, I focused on the relief that I would undoubtedly feel at the end of the first trimester. One morning I awakened, nearly eight weeks along, and the cloud was instantly lifted. I felt energetic and alive. Overnight, my stomach transformed from a massive catapult into an industrial strength vacuum as it demanded to be filled and re-filled. How fortunate that my pregnancy, and undoubtedly my baby as well, was so precocious that it advanced right past the difficult stage four weeks earlier than average! If I kept it up at this rate, the baby would surely come out changing its own diapers!

The night before my first ultrasound appointment, James and I sat marveling at the small, but noticeable bump poking its way out of my abdomen.

"We're going to see you tomorrow," James spoke tenderly to my belly. "We'll have our first little piece of your baby album."

I smiled, thinking about the fuzzy little blobs that ultrasounds displayed. I was sure that our little blob was going to be awfully cute.

"I hope that you look like Dada," I chimed into the conversation with the fetus, "But let's try to keep your head at a reasonable size." I winced at the thought of having to deliver James' head.

"We should take a picture of your belly each week to see how it changes." James suggested. He wrote "8 ½ weeks" on a piece of paper. "Here, hold this next to the baby."

"Smile baby," James said as he snapped the photo, the first piece of physical evidence of our precious little one.

James and I arrived at the obstetrician's office in the middle of the morning. After filling out a mound of first-visit paperwork, we sat in the waiting room. I picked up a random baby magazine and thumbed through it.

"Do you want to use a diaper service?" I asked James as I glanced at a Tiny Tot's advertisement, "Or do you think we could handle washing the diapers on our own?"

"I don't know," James replied. "We'll have to look into how much it costs."

"Look at this article," I shoved the magazine toward James, "Did you know that we could have the baby's cord blood saved in case it gets sick later in life?"

"I haven't heard of that, but it sounds like a good idea," James responded.

Clearly there was a lot of research that we still needed to do before this baby came! I continued to skim and jot mental notes until the sound of my name jolted me out of my seat. Throwing down the magazine, I grasped James' hand and followed the nurse to the exam room.

When the doctor came in, she sat down and we started to chat. Dr. Jackman was a middle-aged woman with a gentle smile and a pleasant demeanor. My method for choosing a doctor had been to pick the one who offered the earliest possible appointment. I had no idea if she was any good at what she did. The books that I had been reading suggested that you interview the doctor on the first visit to make sure that his or her philosophies are in line with yours. So I proceeded to ask her about episiotomies, C-sections, pain management, and every delivery-related topic I could come up with. She seemed like a reasonable person.

After our chat, we went ahead with the pelvic exam. I noticed that I felt a bit awkward having a doctor examine me in front of James. This would take some getting used to. After the exam, we finally got to the point we had been waiting for. As Dr. Jackman wheeled the ultrasound machine over, my heart started racing. We were finally going to catch a glimpse of the little being growing inside! She began the ultrasound, facing the screen toward her. Frustrated that I couldn't see anything, I fixed my eyes on her face, waiting for the slight nod or smile which would indicate that she had located our little peanut. Her expression betrayed nothing, and she remained silent. I wondered how long it was supposed to take to find a baby at this stage on an ultrasound. I took a deep breath and squeezed James' hand. Silence continued to fill the room. Finally Dr. Jackman spoke.

"I'm concerned about the size of the baby," she said in a monotone.

The four walls of the room started pressing in around me. The dense mass of air above me rested heavily on my chest.

"Take a look." The doctor turned the screen of the ultrasound machine toward me. The sound of her voice was muffled as it worked its way through the thick space.

"At this stage in pregnancy, we would expect to see a much larger baby. We would see the little flicker of a heartbeat."

I sank deeper into the table. My eyes glazed over as I stared at the screen.

"Also, take a look at the sac. You would expect it to be round, but it appears to be beginning to collapse."

I stared at my baby whose world was literally crashing in around it. *This can't be happening.*

"I think that this is a miscarriage."

A miscarriage? This is not how miscarriages happen!

From what I had seen on TV, miscarriages always came dramatically, with bleeding and intense cramping. How could my body have had a miscarriage without me knowing it?

"Are you sure about this?" James asked, clutching my hand.

"I want to do a blood test today and then repeat the same test in two days to confirm that the hormone levels are no longer doubling." Dr. Jackman paused, "I don't want to do anything until I am sure."

"What do you mean?" I asked. "What would we do?"

"Well, we could wait for your body to naturally expel the pregnancy or we could do a procedure called a D&C, where we remove the contents of the uterus using suction." She paused, "But let's just wait for the test results."

I silently got dressed. James and I walked to the lab, eyes unfocused, minds unable to grasp what we had just experienced. After the lab technician had collected from my arm the evidence to build the doctor's case against our baby, we headed home.

Returning home, we collapsed into bed and sobbed in each other's arms. We cursed the heavens for our inability to shore up the collapsing walls of our baby's little sac home, our inability to see or hold our child who was experiencing death before life. How could this be happening after all that we'd gone through to bring this baby into existence? What did we do wrong to deserve this?

I honestly don't remember anything about the ensuing two days of limbo as we waited for the second blood test. We had been sucked into a black hole where we clung to each other, hiding from the world, willing our brains into a state of paralysis. On Wednesday, when the doctor called about the results of the second blood test, I reluctantly answered the phone and braced for the inevitable bad news.

"The hormone levels are still doubling," Dr. Jackman sounded baffled. "I'd like to wait until Monday to do a follow-up ultrasound to see if there has been any growth."

Are you serious? Five more days of half-existence?

"Is there any chance that the baby is OK?" I asked, recalling the image of the lifeless lump in its collapsing sac.

"Well, it's very unlikely, but I just want to be sure."

I made an appointment for Monday and hung up, but the doctor's indecisive tone bothered me.

"I think we should get a second opinion." I said to James.

So on Thursday, we returned to the scene of the emotional carnage that had taken place days earlier. This time, I averted my eyes from the baby magazines. I tried to tune out the happy sounds of the couples, exiting with pictures of the healthy contents of their bulging, life-filled wombs.

Entering the exam room, I winced at the sight of the ultrasound machine which had coldly announced the death of our dreams. Dr. Gravel strutted in and got straight to business. He expertly located the baby, even as the screen faced us.

"There is no question in my mind that this is a miscarriage," he said unemotionally. "There has been no growth since Dr. Jackman's ultrasound, and at almost nine weeks, it is unheard of to not see a heartbeat."

"But what about the fact that the hormone levels are still doubling?" James asked.

"That is very common. Sometimes it takes a while for the body to realize what has happened. But look, this is a really common thing. One in six pregnancies end in early miscarriage. It is nature's system of quality control. This thing wasn't even a baby. It's not going to heaven or anything. It is just some genetic mistake." He must have noticed the shock on our faces at the way he was speaking. "Don't worry. You're young. You'll be back here before the year is out delivering a healthy baby."

Although this guy was about as sensitive as a bulldozer, at least he was confident in what he was saying. We decided to go ahead with the D&C which we scheduled for the next day with Dr. Jackman.

I had been prescribed a suppository to take a couple of hours before the procedure which was supposed to soften and open up the cervix. The suppository did its job, and by the time we arrived for the procedure, I had started to bleed and was experiencing severe cramping. So there we sat in the bastion of bulging bellies, waiting to have our baby forcibly vacuumed out of my body. Having witnessed enough of my writhing, James approached the reception desk and pleaded.

"My wife is in so much pain. Isn't there a place where she could lie down and wait for the doctor?"

"I'm sorry, sir," the receptionist didn't even look up to respond. "We don't have any rooms open."

What kind of a sick clinic was this that would place women experiencing the excruciating evacuation of their hopes and dreams in the same room with these blissful women, contentedly sitting, stroking their disgusting, lucky bellies?

A nurse finally called me in, but this time James didn't get to accompany me. I was led into a room where I saw a large machine and various tools lined up in a sterile row. I felt like a prisoner of war surveying the instruments of my impending torture. As I placed my legs into the stirrups, Dr. Jackman and her nurse started the prep for the procedure.

"Will I be getting anesthesia?" I asked, desperately hunting for an escape from this experience.

"We'll just do a local," Dr. Jackman replied. "You shouldn't feel any pain."

Not even a valium to spare for me, eh?

Soon the room was filled with the roar of the vacuum machine. I listened to the sucking sounds of the womb demolition. Clear tubes were delivering blood and tissue into a clear container. Contrary to what had been promised, the pain was indescribable.

"I can feel that!" I whimpered. "It really hurts!"

"Just keep breathing," the nurse said, with a hint of annoyance in her tone.

If I had been harboring any national secrets, I would have spilled them in an instant if it would have made that pain stop. But as the nurse said, my only option was to breathe. So for the next 15 minutes, my breath stiffly came and went. Every muscle in my body was tightly compressed as I struggled to keep myself from jumping off the table with every stab of pain. At last, the ravenous vacuum fell silent. My baby and its inadequate lodging had been laid to rest in a jar.

As I recovered from the D&C, my sincere wish was to be left completely alone. I fantasized about moving to a new town where no one knew me. I dreaded the gauntlet of pity I would walk through as I faced the countless people who knew about my colossal failure at becoming a mother. To make things worse, my younger cousin Claire, who also worked at my company, was five months pregnant. I imagined the sting of watching her abdomen grow day by day, forcing a smile at her baby shower, congratulating her when she held her healthy baby in her arms, all the while flashing back to my baby's glass jar grave. James and I started browsing the internet for real estate listings in Sacramento and even the Philippines.

The logical side of me knew that it would be a bad idea to make a major life decision such as moving during a time of extreme grief, so James and I decided to take a short vacation instead and revisit the idea of moving when our minds returned to a more rational state. Our first wedding anniversary was only days away, so even though we didn't feel like celebrating, it seemed a good excuse to escape for a while.

James and I checked into a cozy hotel in Carmel for the celebration of our first year of marriage. The tear-stained, swollen-eyed wife on James' arm was the only resemblance to our honeymoon which now felt like a lifetime ago.

We dragged our heavy hearts to the nearby beach. I stepped gingerly on the sand to avoid feeling the residual tenderness from the D&C. The sun was shining brightly, but the strong wind kept our jackets firmly on. Sitting down in the warm sand, we surveyed our surroundings. To our surprise, the beach was overflowing with dogs. Some were leaping over waves to fetch sticks for their owners. Others were exuberantly running at top speed at the water's edge, tails wagging and tongues flapping. James and I smiled for the first time watching these carefree creatures.

"Wouldn't it be nice if we could get that excited over a stick?" I lamented. "That would make our problems seem much smaller."

"Well I could throw one out there for you and see how it goes," James smiled.

I rested my head on his shoulder. "I wish I could just forget that I have this desire," I said, longing for my deepest wish to be for something simple like a rawhide. James nodded and nudged aside the tear that was making its way down my cheek.

"We'll keep trying."

I thought about the nine months of trying that led up to this fiasco. How could we start this agonizing process all over? How long would it take us to conceive again? And then once we did, would recent history repeat itself? Could we really bear opening ourselves up to all of that pain again? I had to ask myself the question even though it already had an answer that must have been hard coded into my brain while I was forming in my mother's womb. Of course we would try again and again – as long as it took to succeed.

Chapter 4
Fortune Cookie Fever

Our Carmel trip came to an end, and we were forced to return to reality. It was time to face all of the people whom we had been avoiding. All of our friends and loved-ones had a great deal of sympathy for what we had been through and wanted to support us in every way possible. Unfortunately, there is no rulebook for how to comfort someone who is recovering from a miscarriage. A rulebook could never exist because every person experiencing this kind of a tragedy would respond differently to different forms of comfort. I was in a very angry place at the time, so I was polite on the outside but highly unreceptive on the inside to most people's attempts at comfort. After a little while, I began to observe that most people's responses to my situation broke down into three basic categories.

1) Awkward Silence. This is when someone would approach me, sheepishly say "hello," maybe "how are you," and then silently fidget as they waited for me to say something to break the excruciating tension of the moment. Usually I would fend this one off by quickly turning the topic to the other person's life. The person would then be satisfied (and exceedingly relieved) that I didn't want to talk about my ordeal. A hasty update from the person would be followed by a swift exit. Not too terribly painful.

2) The Fortune Cookie Response. This refers to the natural urge people have to respond to the pain of

others by dispensing sunny predictions or shiny pearls of wisdom. For me, this was the most common and the most irritating response. Below are some examples of the fortune cookies which James and I more commonly swallowed....

    a. "Just you wait. By this time next year, you'll have your baby!" I should have taken this as encouragement, like it was intended. But I found these statements made my inner dialogue turn quite sarcastic, "Gee, I thought nine months of trying followed by a miscarriage was a really bad sign, but if you say so, I'm sure that everything will turn out perfect really soon! What a relief! Thanks so much for bringing me up to speed on my future!" The people making these unfounded predictions weren't doctors, psychics, or prophets, so there was absolutely no basis for what they were saying. They might as well have been telling me my grandfather would soon spring from his grave.

    b. "It will happen when God wills it to happen." Nothing like references to God to get my blood boiling. So He's the one responsible for all of my misery? Why does He not will this to happen? Is it because I'm not worthy enough for a child yet? I've seen some pretty unworthy people who are able to shoot out babies like candy from a Pez dispenser, so I wonder what I could have done to be more unworthy than them. Or is God just randomly messing with our lives like a twisted writer of a soap opera - it was between killing my baby and the surfacing of my evil twin. The baby thing seemed like it would bring in better ratings. God's "plan" always sends you tumbling head-first down a slippery slope. Did

God plan the Holocaust? Is He the mastermind behind the babies who starve to death on a daily basis in Africa? He just didn't *will* them to eat yet? If we believe that of our Higher Power, then I wonder if we may be unintentionally worshipping Satan.

c. "This is nature's special method of quality control." Can you imagine saying that to the mother of a 10 year old who dies of a terminal illness? I wonder why it is OK to say that when the baby has not been born yet. Yes, there may have been something intrinsically weaker about my baby, but should I be relieved that the baby died for the sake of the survival of the species? The thought that we are all just helpless victims of nature's cruel indifference doesn't give me a warm, fuzzy feeling inside. However, I must say that this statement was still vastly more comforting than the image of God purposely inflicting all of the pain for the sake of some unknown "higher purpose."

d. "It's good that it happened early. It would have been a lot worse to have a second or third trimester loss or to lose a baby who's already been born." For every unimaginably bad thing that could happen to a person, I could name at least a dozen ways in which it could have been worse. Is that supposed to make what happened any easier? When for several weeks after the D&C, I would still suddenly and painfully pass large chunks of tissue that had accidentally been left behind in my death-scene uterus, I would chuckle and say, "At least I wasn't beheaded with a chainsaw today. Lucky that didn't happen." It actually turned into a running joke between James and me, and even though the statements themselves didn't provide comfort for us, the humor we found in it was quite therapeutic.

3) This Really Stinks Big Time Response. This was the response which resonated the most for me personally. I was seriously pissed off that something this terrible could happen to me. When people stood alongside me in my outrage, it was incredibly validating. I didn't want to hear that the event which was causing me to wake up in a puddle of tears every morning was some kind of a blessing in disguise. I wanted to hear that it was the highest degree possible of wrong and unfair.

So for several weeks, James and I endured the awkward encounters here and there. We tolerated the processed cookie sweetness lingering in our mouths. We leaned on the people we were closest to, who more often than not were in the "This Really Stinks" club. After a few weeks, the spotlight on us was finally dimming. Interactions started to feel normal again. My pillow was even getting scattered reprieves from its daily dampening sessions. My mind started making the gradual turn from grief mode into planning mode. It was time dust ourselves off and try again.

We had been told to wait one full cycle after the miscarriage before attempting to get pregnant again. As was the new norm for us, even this cycle of wait could not be without drama. After I finally finished passing all of the leftover tissue from the D&C, I started to feel like things had returned to normal. It was right at that point that my relief was rescinded by a burning, itchy irritation which sent me reluctantly back to the doctor. Diagnosed with a rather nasty case of bacterial vaginosis, I began a course of antibiotics. Despite the medication, the infection got worse with each passing day as did my level of anxiety. My frantic mind imagined that a virulent strain of bacteria had been introduced to my uterus from some non-sterile instrument used during the D&C. Probably by now a massive infection was eating its way through all of my insides, consuming the tiny morsel of fertility I had to begin with. The doctor prescribed a round of a different antibiotic which also was no match for the infection. I graduated from pills to antibiotic gel, plunged directly into the site of the infection. Luckily, this course of antibiotics was the one to tip the scales toward me and against the bugs. The infection finally cleared up.

At last I was back to normal, not that normal was anything to celebrate. Normal was a step back in time to face yet again the seemingly endless loop of trying and failing that I had been iterating through for the past year. Each passing cycle, a fresh 40-day round of torment. Even the length of my cycles, almost twice that of a typical cycle, worked against me. And this time, a new pregnancy would not bring the unbridled joy of the first, but rather a new set of worries. The light at the end of my tunnel was on a reverse course, slipping further from my view.

Chapter 5
I'll Meet You in the Morning

For James and me, the pivotal events in our lives often seemed to be accompanied by fireworks. In 2001, James and I had a terrible fight which actually resulted in a brief breakup. This blowup occurred on July 4th amid thunderous explosions both figurative and literal. In 2002, the triumphant return home from our engagement trip was regally announced with the aforementioned, well-timed fireworks display. So it was only fitting that the occasion of our second positive pregnancy test was also marked with 4th of July pyrotechnics. Yes, despite my fears of never being able to get pregnant again, we were successful on our very first try after the miscarriage. As James and I stared blankly at the faint little blue line, we wondered whether we should feel relieved or terrified.

"It must be a good sign that we were able to get pregnant so quickly this time." I reasoned, "Maybe this means that whatever was going wrong has been squared away."

"Yeah, well the doctors all said that the first one was just a fluke." James was correctly quoting the doctors, but I could tell in his tone that I wasn't the only one who was struggling to believe in the fluke theory.

"The best thing we can do for ourselves and the baby is to think positively." I was attempting to convince myself as much as James. "Do you want to tell anyone?"

"Let's keep it to ourselves this time. Just close family."

So the news of our second baby's existence was quietly released to a select few. This time, screams of jubilation were absent from the other end of the phone, replaced with reassurance delivered with unsure tones. The time of unqualified excitement and blissful ignorance was over. And the three-week wait for the deliberation of our ultrasound jury felt like a waterless walk through the desert toward a barely visible speck at the edge of the horizon.

Trying again after the initial disaster, my mind was constantly looking for ways to contrast the second experience from the first. I figured the more different the two experiences were, the more likely the outcome would be different as well. The first obvious difference was that I had gotten pregnant much easier this time. In addition, I was physically feeling considerably better in this pregnancy. I still had food aversions and bouts of nausea, but nothing like the constant state of malaise that I had experienced the first time. I started to accept the theories my mind was pushing that this time was different, and everything was going to be OK. James and I let the news slip out here and there to more people. I held the ultrasound appointment in my mind as the point at which we could finally relax. We would see the heartbeat, and from then on, everything would be fine.

Of course time, in its usual stubborn fashion, became more unwilling to drag itself forward the more I wanted it to proceed. If I could have climbed up on the clock and forced the revolution of the hour hand, I would have. My cousin Claire was getting closer to her due date. I attended her multiple baby showers, grateful that at least I was given the grace of my own pregnancy, however tenuous it was, to dampen the agony.

Finally, the date of the ultrasound arrived. Unable to return to the scene of the first miscarriage, I had made an appointment with a different doctor at a different location. The drive was a bit longer, but we were relieved to be making a fresh start. Music from the band Keane was filling the car with words that fit the moment perfectly: "If only I don't suffocate, I'll meet you on the other side. I'll meet you in the light. If only I don't bend and break, I'll meet you in the morning when you wake." I thought about what was awaiting us at this new doctor's office. Would it bring the long awaited light of morning, or would it bend us deeper into uncharted contortions?

The office had a more warm and pleasant feel to it than the previous one. Still, we had to wade through a sea of bobbing bellies, but we held our breath and made it to our seats. The only available reading material was either related to pregnancy or babies, so we clutched each other's hand and sat blankly. When it was our turn, a young nurse named Barbara, with kind eyes and a cheerful smile, led us to the exam room. She took my blood pressure and then started the standard list of questions.

"Is this your first pregnancy?" She looked up at me and immediately saw my expression dissolve.

"No," I tried to hold back the tears, but they would have no more of being restrained within my troubled head. "The first one was a miscarriage." I barely got the words out as distress took temporary control of my body. With the swiftness of a seasoned shoulder-to-cry-on, Nurse Barbara, in a single move had a tissue in my hand and her hand on my shoulder.

"Oh, I'm so sorry Sweetie," she said with true compassion in her voice. "We'll just skip right past all the other stuff and get that ultrasound machine in here right away."

"Thank you so much." James said, relieved to be spared the cold indifference of the previous clinic.

Not more than a couple minutes later, Dr. Montana was wheeling in the ultrasound machine. A middle aged man with olive complexion and dark, wildly curly hair, he walked in with a confident stance and a jovial expression.

"We'll get this ultrasound out of the way for you really quickly." He said prepping the wand of the machine. We watched the screen as he navigated his way toward our baby. He expertly located the gestational sac. I squinted my eyes as I scanned the sac for some small flicker to indicate a beating heart. Dr. Montana started quietly doing some measurements. The silence in the room carried the now familiar message of dread. James and I had a sinking feeling that this ultrasound was not going to bring us the relief that we so desperately wanted.

The doctor's powerful voice broke the silence, "Well, the baby is measuring around five weeks, six days."

"Is there a heartbeat?" James braced himself for the answer.

"I don't see a heartbeat, but we wouldn't see one anyway at five weeks." Dr. Montana responded.

"But we're not five weeks. We're seven weeks." I said, my heart sinking.

"Well, it's possible that you could be a bit off on your dates." Dr. Montana said calmly, "We have no way of knowing when the fetus actually implanted. We'll do a blood test today and two days from now to check the hormone levels. Also, you can set an appointment to come back in a couple of days for a follow-up ultrasound."

I felt the familiar numbness enveloping my body. There was no chance that I was off on the dates. I was 7 weeks along, and this was not going to be OK.

"This happens quite commonly," Dr. Montana tried to reassure us, "Over half the time, we look again in a couple of days, and we see growth and a heartbeat."

The déjà vu overwhelmed us as we trudged over to the lab and then home to surrender to the black hole that was poised to swallow us. We waited two days for the follow-up lab and ultrasound, which confirmed what we already knew. We were losing another baby.

This time, I was determined to get to the bottom of what was going on with me. I desperately looked to Dr. Montana for some answers. "Now that this has happened twice, we know that it isn't just bad luck, right?"

"Well statistics say otherwise," Dr. Montana replied vehemently, "Even after two miscarriages, the probability of having a third is the same as the probability of the average woman having a single miscarriage. It is not until after a third miscarriage that the odds of repeating go up, and even then, it is still highly likely that the next pregnancy will go to term."

I was completely unconvinced by his explanation. I was only 28 years old. Since the probability of having a single miscarriage for women of all ages is only 1 in 6, the probability of having two in a row by random chance was 1 in 36, or 2.7% - how unlucky could I possibly be? I was awestruck that this man of science could believe what he was telling us. "I don't want to wait to have a third miscarriage to get to the bottom of this." I replied with equal forcefulness. "Are there any tests that you can do now to find out what's wrong with me?"

"Yes, there is a large battery of tests." Dr. Montana replied, "We typically don't perform these tests until after a woman has miscarried three times, but I'd be happy to do the tests for you now."

It astounded me that doctors could require a woman to go through this hell three times before performing simple tests to find out what was wrong. But as long as he was willing do the tests on me now, I was satisfied. We would finally be getting some answers. "Yes, I would like to have the tests done as soon as possible."

"Ok, we'll set that up right away," Dr. Montana assured me. "But before we do the tests, we need to make some decisions about this pregnancy. Do you want to have a D&C or just wait to miscarry naturally?"

My mind flashed back to the gory scene with Dr. Jackman and Nurse Nasty. The last thing I wanted was to go through that again.

"The last D&C was so painful," I said, my voice quivering with the sting of the memory.

"Well, last time you were almost nine weeks along. There was considerably more tissue to remove. This time it will be really fast and easy." Dr. Montana's confidence was convincing. I did want to move on from this pregnancy as quickly as possible. I had heard that some women wait months before passing the pregnancy naturally, and it can be an extremely painful and prolonged process. Plus if all of the tissue doesn't pass naturally, some women end up getting a

D&C anyway after all that. There was no easy way out no matter how I looked at it.

"Ok, I'll go with the D&C." I cringed as the words escaped my lips.

Fortunately, Dr. Montana didn't ask me to use the suppository that had sent my uterus into a state of frenzy prior to the first D&C. Unfortunately, contrary to what I had been promised, the D&C itself was every bit as painful as the first one. The only consolation was that Nurse Barbara was there, coaching me through it and encouraging me the entire time. Seeing in my face every wince of pain, she squeezed my hand tightly and gently repeated the mantra, "You're doing great. We're almost done."

Finally it was done. James helped me to the car with his strong arm around my waist. We drove home in silence. The morning light that we desperately longed to see was still being held hostage just beyond the horizon. And no amount of praying, pleading, bargaining or wishing could release it into our view. I wondered how long a person could take being starved of morning. Was this deprivation going to eventually break us?

Chapter 6
The Stranger

Since getting away after the first miscarriage had been quite helpful for us, James and I left for a short trip to Monterey the day after the D&C. Seeking maximum distraction, we ventured out to the Monterey Bay Aquarium. Wanting to limit my exertion so soon after the surgery, James insisted that I sit in a wheelchair during our visit. I felt like I was physically well enough to get around on my own, but I went along with it since he was very concerned about setting back my recovery. Moving around in a wheelchair was a new experience for me. I felt like an imposter since I wasn't actually handicapped in the usual sense of the word – they don't give out handicapped placards to the infertile. In front of one display, I found myself next to a woman about my age who was legitimately in a wheelchair. I tried not to make eye contact, since she would probably be able to tell immediately by some sort of radar that I was not an authentic handicapped person. I started wondering if she was able to sustain a pregnancy. I figured she probably was since it looked like it was just her legs that were the problem. Immediately, I thought about trading places with her. I would accept any disability if it would mean that I could experience pregnancy and childbirth. I had often bargained with God in this way asking Him to give me any other sort of cross to bear. It would be worth it if I could have the experience of motherhood that I so desperately wanted.

Cheerful cooing sounds interrupted my train of thought. I looked up and saw a chubby-cheeked baby girl, around five months old, gazing in amazement at the colorful array of sea life in front of us. She stared with wide eyes, her gaping mouth turned up in a slight smile. Her legs excitedly kicked from underneath the front pack securing her to her mother. James and I had often talked about bringing our children to the aquarium from little on and fostering in them a love of nature. To me, it almost seemed like the displays weren't worth seeing except through the eyes of a child. I gazed into the tank and my eyes started to follow a yellow-fin tuna. *Well, you may be in captivity, but probably even you have no trouble reproducing.* It struck me that life had brought me to a point so low that I would seriously envy a fish.

  After visiting the aquarium, we checked into a charming bed and breakfast in Pacific Grove which had been the home of a Senator back in the 1800s. Walking into our room, we felt like we were stepping back in time. Purple floral wallpaper set against ornate crown moldings lined the walls of the small room. In one corner stood a beautiful white claw-footed bathtub with a lace curtain surrounding it, suspended directly above. A large, wood-paneled, antique radio sat on a small side table alongside the bed. This elegant, old-fashioned setting, so different from what we were used to, filled us with a welcome feeling of transcendence. We snuggled in the frilly bed and listened to an old-style radio mystery program. For a brief moment, we were some other couple in some other time with some other set of problems that were certainly much less distressing than ours.

  I returned to work early on my first day back after the miscarriage. I figured it would be easier to acclimate myself before others arrived than it would be to make a conspicuous entrance. Upon arriving, I marched directly to the coffee station to rebelliously break my caffeine restriction. I figured I had earned a bit of a pick-me-up. While I was setting up the coffee-maker, a coworker I didn't know very well came by and started cleaning out her oatmeal bowl.

  "No baby?" She said to me with raised eyebrows.

  I was dumbfounded! How would she even know about the baby? We had kept it pretty quiet this time around. Plus to reopen such a fresh wound seemed so cruel. Then I realized, of course, she *didn't* know about my baby. She was talking about my cousin, Claire, who by this point had passed her due date.

"No, not yet." I replied and made a quick exit to avoid any further discussion.

It wasn't but a few more days, though until Claire delivered her healthy baby girl. I felt terrible that I couldn't just be happy for her, but if I could be jealous of a procreating fish, I figured humans were that much worse. When James, Marsha and I went to visit the new baby, I felt like I was outside of my body watching a character from a movie. The person I saw was holding her cousin's beautiful baby, but had no sense of joy and wonder at the new life. This stranger was nothing like me. I was the person who preferred to hang out with the babies at parties over the adults. I was the person who would smile at the sight of a baby no matter how low my mood was. I was the person who would call dibs on changing my nieces' and nephews' diapers just so I could get the chance to care for them. This woman was someone I didn't understand and didn't like. I wondered if this bitter, lost soul who had taken over my body would ever leave, or if I would have to coexist with her for the rest of my life.

Chapter 7
Failure to Flunk

When I was in school, I had a serious problem with perfectionism. I didn't just want to pass my classes, I wanted to ace every single one of them. It was not uncommon for a B+ to elicit both pain and panic. But now, as the lab technician was drawing the 13 vials of blood for my miscarriage panel, I was praying with all my might that I would fail at least one of the tests. We couldn't fix what was wrong if we didn't know what it was.

A few weeks after my massive blood donation, I got a call from Dr. Montana.

"All your test results have come in," Dr. Montana said, "And I'd like to go over them with you. Do you have some time now?"

"Yes, definitely," I responded. That sounded promising. If there was something to "go over," maybe he had found the problem.

Dr. Montana proceeded to go through each and every test. Genetic karyotype – normal for both James and me. A slough of hormonal tests – normal. Thrombophilia panel – normal. The only slight blip was a heterozygous positive for the MTHFR gene 1928A, which Dr. Montana said was meaningless since over 40% of the population had this mutation, and it was only an issue when it was homozygous.

"Are you sure those are all the tests that we can do?" I questioned, desperately hoping there might be a second panel for those who found nothing in the first panel.

"We've done all of the tests that exist to identify problems associated with miscarriage." Dr. Montana definitively stated. Sensing my disappointment, he added, "This is great news. It means that these two pregnancies have almost certainly been chromosomal problems with the baby, which happen from time to time due to random chance. You were just unlucky enough to have it happen twice in a row."

My gut knew that it was not that simple. "What about my difficulty getting pregnant the first time? What about my long cycles?"

"Studies have shown no link between long menstrual cycles and miscarriage." Dr. Montana assured me, "But if you have trouble getting pregnant again, you can come back, and I will be happy to help you along with some medications."

I did feel slightly reassured by that promise. At least if we had difficulty getting pregnant again, we would not be totally on our own. But I was nearly certain that my babies had been normal and that there was something wrong with me. I realized that this might have been outside of Dr. Montana's expertise. Probably nine times out of ten, his job was to deliver normal babies of normal women. As soon as I hung up the phone, I searched the internet for a specialist. I saw that the High Risk ObGyn group at Stanford did consults for people who had recurrent miscarriage. I called them and set up an appointment.

As I sat in the consult with Dr. Lionel at Stanford, my shoulders became increasingly slumped with each passing minute. She was echoing Dr. Montana practically verbatim. I wondered if all of the doctors were sharing the same manual for <u>How to Snow a Miscarriage Sufferer</u>. She said that a woman wasn't even considered to have recurrent miscarriage until she has had three in a row. She again offered up the statistic of my 68% chance of going to term with my next pregnancy without doing any sort of treatment. But then she deviated from the script for a moment, and my ears perked up. There was one test which had not been done yet – a hysteroscopy. In this procedure, the doctor inflates the uterus with fluid and then examines it using a camera. This is done to simultaneously identify and treat structural abnormalities in the uterus that can lead to miscarriage. I asked Dr. Lionel to sign me up right away.

On the day of the hysteroscopy, James and I arrived at the hospital around 6:00 am. After filling out several forms and releasing the hospital from any and all liability, I got in my gown and settled into a cozy bed with blankets that had just been nicely warmed. The anesthesiologist placed my IV, and I was already hearing the gentle lullaby of the anesthesia as the team wheeled me into the operating room. The lights faded, and soon everything was dark.

"Julie, wake up." The surgeon was standing over me. It seemed like no time had passed, but it was clear that the procedure was over. Even in my groggy state, my heart started to race in anticipation of the news. *Please God, let her tell me that I flunked this test. Let her tell me that she fixed the problem while she was in there.*

"The procedure went well." The surgeon continued, "I saw a little bit of scarring around the cervix, which was probably due to the D&C's, but other than that, everything looked perfect."

I think the doctor was expecting me to be relieved, but tears immediately started pooling in my groggy, unfocused eyes. This was the most painful blow that I had received since the last ultrasound. A uterine abnormality had been my last hope of an explanation for my pregnancy disasters. With that hope gone, there was nothing to do but blindly try again, with very little confidence that the next try would be any different from the first two.

Chapter 8
Superstitions

When science fails you, the next natural step is to turn to superstition. James and I went over every detail that we could think of. Could we have jinxed ourselves by telling people about the pregnancies too soon? Was there someone we had told who secretly had negative thoughts about our babies that had adversely affected the pregnancies? Was this happening because I was resenting pregnant women so much that I had actually placed some sort of a curse on myself? I started to police my thoughts in an effort to eradicate my disgust of the ease at which others reproduced. This was a tall order for me, but I hoped that whatever force may have placed this curse might at least recognize my effort to improve. I started a campaign to ensure that my karma was intact. I was very careful not to step on any bugs. If I found a spider in the house, I would painstakingly catch it and release it outside. I recycled everything properly and bought reusable grocery bags, produce bags, and sandwich bags. I made sure that I bought only cage-free eggs, organic produce, and fair-trade products whenever possible. These things had always been important to me, but now I was taking it to a new level of obsession. I feared that if I faltered in any way in maintaining the utmost respect for life and the earth, the powers that be might have a reason to take something more out on my children.

The other possibility which occurred to James and me was that there was some sort of chemical in our house that was silently poisoning our unborn children. This thought propelled us to revisit the idea of moving. At that time, the market for condos and townhouses in our area was soaring, so we figured it would actually be a great opportunity for us to get into a single family home. We loved our townhouse, but the idea of having a nice yard for our kids and dogs to run around in was very appealing. Getting excited about something new would have the added benefit of temporarily diverting our attention from fertility struggles.

After about a week of looking, we found the perfect house. It was a single level home on a quiet, well-kept street. It originally had four bedrooms, but two of them had been combined to make a spacious master bedroom with ample room for an office. The entire house was covered in beautifully restored hardwood floors except for the dining room, which had plush carpeting. The kitchen, though small and outdated, was still bigger than the kitchen we had in the townhouse, and it had an adorable little breakfast nook. The attached garage was constructed in a really cute barn style. And the best thing was that above the garage, the attic space had been converted to a room. A small spiral staircase led up to the *secret room* which had built-in cabinets on three walls and a large work surface on the fourth. James and I figured this room could make a great music studio. We also pictured Marsha having slumber parties and spending time with her friends doing school projects up in the secret room. This house was absolutely perfect! We had to have it. Knowing that the housing market was crazy at the time, we bid $15,000 over the asking price, which was the absolute maximum that our tight budget would stretch.

On the following Friday, the seller's agent presented the offers. I anxiously waited for a phone call from my realtor. The phone seemed to have taken a vow of silence for the entire day. I repeatedly checked it to make sure that it was still working. Finally, by 6:00 in the evening, I couldn't take the suspense anymore, and I called him myself.

"Oh hi Julie," Jack answered, "I was just about to call you. I just got off the phone with the seller's agent." Jack cleared his throat and sighed. "They were just about to accept your offer, when right at 5:00, an offer came in for $40,000 over asking. I guess this one just wasn't meant to be."

I slumped down on the couch, and sobbed. So many things lately weren't *meant to be*. Why did we never get the things we wanted – the things that were perfect for us! I felt like a human Jenga game. I kept trying to build something, but as I carefully laid the bricks, someone else was yanking out other ones beneath me, gradually eating away at the foundation. It was only a matter of time before the brick would be pulled that would send the whole structure crashing down.

Jack continued to send me listings when he spotted ones which he thought might interest me. I half-heartedly looked them over, and none of them measured up to my cute little barn with the secret room. One day, Jack called me at work.

"Did you get the listing I sent this morning?" Jack asked, his voice bursting with enthusiasm.

"Yeah, but it has only a one-car garage." I replied flatly.

"Well, I took a look at it this morning, and it's really not a one-car garage. The garage door is the width of one car, but the garage itself is the size of a two-car garage. The house is really great. I think you should take a look at it."

I didn't hold out much hope. But since Jack had gone through all of the effort to check it out, I agreed to take a look on my lunch hour. When I turned onto the street the house was on, I was struck by how charming the neighborhood was. The well-kept tract homes looked like cozy little cottages, resting under a canopy of towering ash trees. The house was equally delightful on the inside. The living room sat behind a beautiful picture window, and beams of light cast the silhouette of the ash tree on the blinds. The good-sized kitchen was recently updated, with a ton of counter space. Past the kitchen was an added-on family room with parquet flooring and a sliding glass door leading out to a small, but pleasant back yard. I pictured our dogs hanging out in that room with access to the yard, but not able to track mud through the entire house. There were four bedrooms, which was ideal for us. Regardless of nature's attempts to deter us, we did intend to have two more children, and it would be nice for all three to have their own room. In the back yard, stepping stones on the grass led the way to a sturdy wooden shed, which the owner had been using as a saddle-making workshop. This shed also had possibilities of being converted into the music studio that James and I had dreamed of. The garage was the size of a two-car garage, as Jack had promised. I hated to admit it, but this house was actually better than my barn house. To top it all off, it was $55,000 cheaper!

I quickly called James, and he came out to take a look. He also fell in love with the house, and we immediately agreed to put an offer on it. We tried to contain our enthusiasm because there was still a high likelihood of being outbid again.

That evening, the phone rang. Jack sounded as though he could barely catch his breath. "I made a call to the seller's agent just to get a feel for things, and she is really eager to wrap this deal up because she is due to have some surgery. I got her to agree to present your offer on Friday, before the open house."

I couldn't believe the luck! If we could get an offer in without any competition, we might actually have a shot at getting the house. So we went for it, and offered $3000 over asking, just for good measure. Friday night, Jack called and delivered our first stroke of good fortune in a long time – our offer had been accepted!!

I thought about how bleak things had seemed when we lost our barn house. But we kept at it and ended up getting something much, much better. I wondered if it was possible for that to happen with our infertility struggle. Could we somehow end up better off when all of this was over? I couldn't really imagine how that could happen. What could possibly be better than the children we had lost? Was there something waiting for us in the future that could make all of the agony worthwhile? It was impossible to fathom, but maybe that was simply because it wasn't over yet.

Chapter 9
Modern Technology

In November of 2004, four days before our first baby's due date, we moved into our new home, ready to make a fresh start. As we settled in, we immediately discovered that we not only had a great house, but we also had extremely friendly neighbors. Even in the busy hub of the Silicon Valley, the people on our street hung out in their front yards and talked to one another. They actually had block parties from time to time, which I had imagined only happened in small towns in the Midwest. It wasn't long before we knew practically everyone on the street, and Marsha had made a couple of friends that were her age. It was clear that we had made the right move. We felt encouraged that maybe this house would not be cursed as the last one was.

But as the months passed, along with many unsuccessful attempts at conceiving, we started to realize that some problems had followed us to the new neighborhood. After eight months of failures, we decided that it was time to take Dr. Montana up on his promise to help us along.

Dr. Montana described for us the various ways that science could intervene on our behalf. Eager to make it happen as quickly as possible, we opted for the complete package – ovarian stimulation followed by a shot of hcg to release the mature eggs, topping it off with intrauterine insemination (IUI) at the optimal time. Dr. Montana prescribed Clomid to give my ovaries the extra push. We followed by ultrasound the development of the follicles which held the maturing eggs in my ovaries, and it soon became clear that the Clomid had produced no effect. My follicles were taking their own sweet time to grow and would not be persuaded otherwise by 50 mg of chemical encouragement. I was headed for another 40-day cycle.

Dr. Montana upped the dosage for the next cycle. I could tell right away that the medicine was having some sort of effect at the increased dosage because my moods had been hijacked and dragged haphazardly from one extreme elevation to another. I would suddenly find my cheeks flushed and stomach queasy, wracked with the distinct feeling of tremendous guilt. I would attempt to recall what reprehensible thing I had done to put me in this state, but I wouldn't be able to come up with anything. Next thing I knew, I would feel extreme panic. My heart and lungs would race each other like an invisible lion was following me around, ready to pounce at any moment. Then the sadness would kick in, and the least little thing would make me cry (even more so than usual, so we're talking some serious waterworks!) I found it so bizarre that feelings could just exist on their own and mill around all over my body without actual events to bring them into being. I hoped that the Clomid was having as much effect on my ovaries as it was having on my brain.

On day seven of my cycle, an ultrasound did confirm what my emotions were shouting – the Clomid had worked at this dosage. I had two large follicles developing in my ovaries on the fast track. Dr. Montana tracked the growth, and when the follicles became large enough, I was instructed to administer a shot of hcg the following evening.

On the day that I was to administer the shot, I waited for evening like a child cowers after hearing the dreaded "Wait til your father comes home." I watched out the front window as the sun departed, leaving me to face my unavoidable punishment. Pulling out the syringe, I prepared the shot. As I stared at the needle, I wondered how it was possible to ignore all of your instincts adamantly warning you that stabbing yourself with a sharp object is generally not a good idea.

I took a pinch of fat on my leg and counted, "One, two, three." My hand refused to plunge the needle into myself. I

Modern Technology

took a deep breath. "One, two, three." Again nothing. After counting to three five or six times, I turned to James.

"I don't think I can do this. You think you can do it for me?"

James calmly nodded, and I quickly forfeited the syringe over to my braver half.

Pinching my thigh, he held the needle steadily over it.

"Ok, on three," James said as I closed my eyes and braced myself. "One, two, three."

Without flinching, he assertively jabbed the needle right in. I was amazed at how confident he was and how little it hurt. His technique was every bit as good as any nurse who had ever given me a shot. I marveled at what an amazing man I had married! His muscular frame had carried so much of the load of our struggles. I had naturally been the focus of most of the sympathy that had come our way through this ordeal since it was my body that had been battered by pregnancy and surgery. But James had suffered every bit as much if not more than I had. At least I had my gentle friend Vicadin to keep me company through the long, dark nights after the D&Cs. James, on the other hand, without benefit of any sedative, had the responsibility of simultaneously caring for a fragile wife and keeping himself sane. Given the choice, I would rather endure physical suffering myself than to have to watch a loved-one in agony. James' steadfast love for me and our future children was solely responsible for preventing my total mental collapse. And the next day, the poor guy would have to ejaculate into a cup and hand it over to the scrutiny of doctors for the cause. Regardless of all my recent failures, I knew that I had done one thing right in my life when I snagged this man.

The following morning, James dutifully made his deposit in the sterile cup. As we drove to Dr. Montana's office, I cradled the cup against my abdomen to keep the little guys at a comfortable body temperature. We delivered the sample on time and then waited as the lab technicians ran it through a centrifuge, cleaned it, and weeded out the duds, leaving only the feistiest swimmers for the job.

Several hours later, James and I entered the exam room and waited for Dr. Montana to arrive with James' sparkling clean Olympic swimmers.

"It will be kind of creepy to conceive our baby with a third party in the room." I remarked.

"Yeah it will," James nodded, "I mean what do we say to the doc when it's over? Was it good for you?"

I almost spit out the water I was sipping. "We just better hope that they bring in the right sperm sample." I thought back to a story I had heard on the news of a doctor who had substituted his own sperm and fathered hundreds of children. "When this baby comes out, it better not have a mop of dark curly hair."

A knock at the door abruptly stifled our chuckling, and Dr. Montana entered, catheter in hand. The procedure was fairly simple. Dr. Montana inserted Team Sperm directly into my uterus, and then instructed me to remain lying down for 20 minutes. When the time was up, we gathered our belongings and departed for another two week wait.

Chapter 10
My Grandfather's Patience

The spring of 2005 cast a warm glow over our new home. Buds began appearing on the plants outside. Not knowing much about gardening, I was pleasantly surprised that many of the plants in our yard produced flowers. I eagerly anticipated the opening of the buds, unveiling the mysterious flowers that were hiding inside. On the bald spot on our back lawn, I had planted some grass seed in the previous week, and the morning after our IUI, tiny green blades began to peak out and stand tall. Of course, I took that as a metaphor of what was going on inside of me – life and growth. Little by little, I began to detect small hints of the now familiar feelings of breast tenderness, exhaustion, and slight nausea. I strongly sensed that there was a new little life unfolding inside of me.

To be sure, I took another pregnancy test two weeks after the IUI, and James and I sat dazed on the bed, once again staring at two solid blue lines. Thus far these lines had only served as precursors to bad news, so we braced ourselves for what was coming. Not long after, the familiar all-day queasiness pushed its way back into my daily routine. I realized right away that this pregnancy was going to be similar to the first in terms of nausea. But as long as the nausea was there, I knew there was something growing inside.

When I was six weeks along, James and I took a short trip to the Sierras to spend some time in the vacation house that my grandfather had built when I was a small child. Breathing the fresh mountain air would do us both some good. "The House in the Country," as my brother had named it when he was four, held cherished childhood memories of romping through the woods with cousins, sledding down the glistening hillside, eating "ice cream" made of snow, and playing board games all through the evening. Grandpa had always dreamed of designing and building his own house in the woods. A sheet-metal worker by trade, he had to wait until he was in his 50's to realize his dream. As soon as it was financially possible, he bought the land and built his dream one nail at a time. Never did his eyes smile more brightly than when he sat on the wrap-around redwood deck peering over a book at his grandchildren gleefully running around his creation. And now it still stood proudly among the pine trees, a monument to Grandpa's love for his family.

It was calming to be in a place so alive with my grandfather's spirit. Sitting back in Grandpa's old recliner, I marveled at how he was able to stay determined and focused on his dream even though it took him practically a lifetime to make it a reality. I believe that I inherited Grandpa's drive and focus, but his gene for patience had skipped over me. This was a bad combination of traits - determination bordering on obsession without the ability to calmly trust in the ultimate outcome. I was like a well-tuned, off-road vehicle, roaring up a cliff side on a hot day with no radiator. As I laid my head on my pillow that evening, I prayed that God would grant me some of my grandfather's patience.

The next morning, the sun burst into the bedroom through the edges of the window shade. I opened my eyes a crack and promptly retreated into the warmth of my pillow; I was not eager to let my stomach know that it was morning, giving it license to assault me once again. Slipping back into the unconscious, my drowsy mind formed a picture of a steaming vegetable omelet smothered with cheese. My mouth watered as I approached it, my grumbling stomach summoning the eggs to the cozy warmth inside. As I eagerly dipped in the fork, my eyes popped open and I sprung up in bed.

Why was I lusting after food? I hadn't had a pleasant thought about food in weeks! I stood up, and walked around a bit, willing my stomach to reel against my sudden movements. But my stomach had no response. I forced into my mind a picture of oily curry and fried fish, visions which one day earlier would have sent me on a mad dash for the nearest container capable of housing vomit. But nothing happened. I felt wretchedly perfect. I felt like I was not pregnant.

On the drive home, as I blankly stared out the window, James could sense my surrender to the powerful strangle of hopelessness.

"We are going to be OK," he said, squeezing my hand.

"How can we ever be OK?" I listlessly muttered, "Why does everything have to be so hard for us? Our life was not supposed to be like this."

"I know," he replied, and paused, trying to hold back the tears which would blur his view of the road. "If this pregnancy ends up…like the others," he squeezed my hand tighter, "What would you think about adopting a baby?" The words hung in the car for a moment before he continued, "We wouldn't have to give up trying to have a biological child, but at least we could start building our family together. And maybe there's a baby out there who needs parents like us."

With his words, James instantly yanked my soul from the dark, slippery tunnel it was spiraling down. Prior to this moment, I had viewed biological children and adopted children as being two mutually exclusive concepts. I had assumed that if and when we finally gave up any hope of having a biological child that we would embrace the idea of adoption and move on from there. The thought of adopting a baby now and continuing to try was extremely appealing. We could finally release all of the love and parental instinct that had been caged up for so long. We could move forward with our lives, and the fertility struggles could be relegated to the background. If we eventually had a biological child, then that would just be icing on the cake.

I mean, I did still desperately want the fundamental experience of creating a life and feeling it grow inside of me. I wanted the experience of childbirth and meeting this little unique piece of myself and the man I love. As much as that experience meant to me, I did know deep down that it was only a fraction of the experience of motherhood. The most important part for me would be what came after the birth - loving and bringing up my children with my husband. I knew firsthand that fact was true because of my beautiful daughter, Marsha. But my experience with Marsha had not been an ideal road to travel. I was still in college and unmarried when Marsha came to live with me. She had severe emotional problems and no language whatsoever at the time. Marsha brought me immeasurable joy from the start, but at the same time, it had been a completely exhausting experience, juggling school and work and a very difficult toddler. I felt like I could never be the mom I wanted to be for her because I had so much other stuff going on as I was just starting my own adult life. By the grace of God, Marsha was actually turning out really well and was a teenager that any parent would dream of having. But I was dying to have the experience of motherhood on my own terms. I wanted my husband and I to bring our infant child home from the hospital before anyone had the chance to harm him or her. I wanted to be a stay-at-home mom with a relaxed schedule and lots of time to explore and learn with my children. I also wanted an excuse to be able to spend more time with Marsha. I couldn't exactly justify quitting work to stay home with a 13-year old who was rarely home herself between school and sports. Adopting a baby would be a way to finally move forward with the life that we were dreaming of.

I threw my arms around James' torso. "You're so right, Sweetie," I replied. "We'll adopt a baby, and we'll keep trying."

Upon returning home from the House in the Country, I called my mom and tearfully told her about my loss of morning sickness. Coming from a long line of optimists, she was positive that there was nothing wrong with the pregnancy.

"Morning sickness comes and goes throughout pregnancy," she said. "You can't draw any conclusions from it."

Doctors had said the same thing to me in the past, but it wasn't as simple as not feeling sick. There was something that I couldn't put my finger on, but remembered from the first pregnancy. I just didn't feel pregnant.

"Mom," I said, "I can just tell that there is something wrong."

"Is there any way you can get in for an ultrasound before Tuesday?" She asked. It was Saturday of a long weekend – you guessed it – 4th of July weekend.

"The clinic won't even be open until Tuesday anyway because of the holiday."

"Then you need to go to the Emergency Room." She stated firmly. "You need to have an ultrasound and see that everything is alright."

I was hesitant to go through hours of waiting in a crowded ER for the opportunity to see another dead baby on an ultrasound. But I am the type of person who would rather have bad news delivered promptly than to linger in a state of fear of the unknown. Plus the thought did occur to me that if by some miracle, Mom was right, and the baby was OK, then it would sure be nice to get some relief from this misery in the near term.

So late that evening, James and I went to the ER and waited several hours for my name to be called. As it turned out, they didn't even have an ultrasound machine in the ER, so all they could really do was take my vitals and perform a blood test to confirm that I was in fact pregnant. But they did say that I could return the next morning for an ultrasound in Radiology. Exhausted, James and I went home and attempted to sleep. With each passing, wakeful hour, I placed all my energy toward erecting a barrier of numbness to hold back the panic at least until I could confirm what was actually happening.

By the morning, I had forced myself into a trance-like state. We drove to the hospital in silence. When it was our turn, I vacantly trudged to the exam room, eyes fixed on thin air. I didn't even bother to look at the screen as the technician performed measurement after measurement. Her silence told an all too familiar story of death and loss. At one point, I started to hear some whooshing sounds like those made by a

Doppler. I wondered why we needed such thorough measurements when all she really needed to do was inform us of the baby's motionless little heart so we could get on with things.

The technician turned from the screen, "Mom's heart rate is 75 beats per minutes, and Baby's is 160."

My conscious mind flew to the forefront and went over that statement again. "There's a heartbeat?" I said.

"Yes, take a look here." The technician turned the screen, and James and I saw a tiny figure with a gloriously flickering little heart! Instantly, both James and I burst into an awkward combination of blubbering and laughter. My legs started to shake uncontrollably in the stirrups. It was actually quite embarrassing – I tried to hold still so the poor technician could complete the ultrasound, but my leg muscles were doing their own little manic jig and would not be interrupted. The patient technician managed to complete the ultrasound despite my hysterics, and James and I left the hospital beaming in disbelief. Our baby was alive and had a vigorously beating heart. Bring on the fireworks!

Despite the miraculous beating heart inside of me, the stress of the previous two days clung to my being like a garment coated with static electricity. I think my body had just not yet caught up with my mind on the huge relief of the successful ultrasound. I kept having to remind myself that there was nothing to worry about. The statistics say that once you see a heartbeat on ultrasound, the odds of carrying to term are over 90%. I tried to focus on the 4th of July festivities to will the uneasy pieces of me into relaxation. As I stared up at the sky filled with color and light, I started to feel my world once again filling with hope. I pictured our little bundle, safe inside, veins coursing with blood. Our family was finally on its way, and come March, we would be too busy as new parents to even remember this two-year blip in our smooth course of happiness.

We still had our regular ultrasound appointment the following day. Having had a successful ultrasound only two days prior, I was feeling a lot more relaxed than I had in a while about a doctor's appointment. I was looking forward to seeing our lively little peanut once again.

When Nurse Barbara called us in, I'm sure she was expecting us to be the uneasy bundle of nerves that we had been the last time. She sympathetically asked, "How are you guys doing?"

"We're doing great," I responded, happy to be able to talk to her without crying for once, "We saw the baby's heart beat two days ago."

I proceeded to tell her the story leading up to our Emergency room visit. She was visibly relieved to hear the good news. "Yes, morning sickness comes and goes," she stated emphatically, "The main symptom at this stage is breast tenderness."

I quickly considered whether my breasts were as tender as they had been. At that moment, Dr. Montana entered the room. We told the ER story once again, and he also seemed very relieved. I'm sure it's no picnic for him to deliver bad news to mothers.

As Dr. Montana began the ultrasound, I found myself unusually chatty.

"It's so amazing how quickly you can navigate around with that ultrasound," I said, watching the screen. "Everything looks the same in there to me."

"Well, when you do this day after day, you can't help but get the hang of it." Dr. Montana responded, smiling, "I couldn't make heads or tails out of the radar images that pilots look at…Ok, here is the sac. Let me zoom in." As the seconds passed, Dr. Montana's smile slowly faded, "Julie, I don't see any heartbeat here. Are you sure that they saw a heartbeat?"

My heart started racing, and my face became flushed.

"Yes, we saw it too." I desperately responded, "We even heard it. It was only two days ago. Couldn't it be hiding behind something else?"

"No, if the heart were beating, we would see it. I'm really sorry."

And with that our third pregnancy ended as mysteriously as the first two. My instinct about my loss of the feeling of pregnancy had been correct. Something had been going terribly wrong. Our timely peek at our little one had been within 48 hours of his or her death.

Before the reality could even sink in, Dr. Montana asked once again about whether or not I wanted a D&C.

"Absolutely not." I sharply replied, "I can't go through that again."

"Well, we could do it in the surgery center under anesthesia if that would make you feel better." Dr. Montana replied.

I couldn't believe that option was there all along and no one ever bothered to mention it! Of course I'd rather be under anesthesia than writhing in pain. I agreed to go forward with the procedure.

I observed Dr. Montana as he wound up the chord of the ultrasound machine, avoiding eye contact with James and me. I cursed myself for listening to him and believing that I could just try again blindly with no treatment.

"Now that we've seen the heartbeat," I addressed Dr. Montana, "We know that this can't be a chromosomal problem with the baby. There is something wrong with me, right?"

"No, there is no reason to draw that conclusion." Dr. Montana responded, "Many times babies with chromosomal problems have beating hearts."

I couldn't believe he was still sticking with that story! "Is there a way that they can check the baby's DNA after the D&C to find out?" I asked.

"I'm not sure," Dr. Montana replied, intrigued at the idea. "I will look into it."

The next day, I underwent my third D&C, but this time resting in the merciful cradle of anesthesia. I felt no physical pain whatsoever, and the drugs even numbed my emotional pain for a time. The exhaustion of this twisted roller coaster ride was overwhelming. I knew that we would not survive if we continued as we were. It was time to move on to adoption.

Chapter 11
Just Adopt

Over the years, I've heard many people say things like, "Well, if things don't work out, we'll just adopt," or "I don't know why those two don't just adopt." I've probably uttered these exact sentences myself in the past. It isn't until you meet this option head-on in your own life that you realize what an oxymoron the phrase "just adopt" is. There is nothing simple or "just" about the process of adoption. In fact, whoever came up with the word "adopt" might have done well to make it a multisyllabic, tongue twister to better capture its meaning. Few things in life place people in a more vulnerable position than that of a prospective adoptive parent. And for the most part, couples who are trying to adopt have already been through the wringer and aren't eager to sign up for more emotional torture.

As I started to consider my options regarding adoption, I drew from knowledge that I had picked up over the years from reading books, watching TV, and talking with people who had adopted children. I knew that there were three basic routes to go with adoption – private adoption, international adoption, and public adoption. Mulling these options over in my head, I could see that they each had their advantages and disadvantages.

International adoption was probably the safest in terms of getting to keep the child. The biological parents would not be able to reclaim their rights from thousands of miles away. In fact, we would probably never even know who the biological parents were. The obvious disadvantages to international adoption for me were the prohibitive cost and the age of the children released for adoption. We'd be lucky to get a child that was under a year old. Part of the experience that I longed for was to have my baby right from the start. So I took international adoption off the table early on.

The costs of public adoption were a clear advantage. However, I knew that to do public adoption, we would have to first take the baby in as a foster child for six months before he or she would be eligible for adoption. During that time, the county could decide to reunify the baby with a biological parent. Or a blood relative could pop up that was willing to take the baby, and we would be out of luck. With all that James and I had been through, I didn't think that we could survive having a baby taken away after bonding with it. Plus with public adoption, the odds are much greater of having a baby who has been exposed to drugs or alcohol in utero, and I knew the long term effects of that could be devastating.

So that only left private adoption. In theory, it seemed like the obvious choice. It would be less costly than international adoption (though still quite costly). We could get more assurances, though never any guarantees, that the biological mother was taking proper care of herself. We would be able to get a newborn baby and possibly even witness the birth. There was still the risk of the birth mother taking back the baby, but at least the wildcard of other relatives popping up in the 11th hour to claim the baby would be mitigated.

So I began to research private adoption on the Internet, first stumbling upon a website of an adoption agency. It said that one of the initial steps for the adoptive parents would be to create a personal statement that birth moms could read in order to begin the selection process. There was a link to actual statements from prospective adoptive parents. I clicked on one of them. Out popped a picture of a smiling couple and their trusty dog in front of a large, immaculate home. Beneath the picture was a detailed resume containing all the reasons that they would make the best parents possible. There were top schools in the neighborhood and great parks. Both members of the smiley couple were active in their church and enjoyed pretty much every outdoor activity possible. They were open to having the birth mom be an important part of the baby's life and saw adoption as a "partnership" with the birth mom. As I read on, my mind flashed a picture of James and me smiling like real estate agents on our personal statement. Beneath the photo would be our painstakingly worded essay in which we would sell ourselves as superior parents. The reader of the essay would be a teenage girl who had everything we ever wanted and complete power over us. We would spend many months presenting an image of perfection to this potentially very immature girl, desperately relying on her to not change her mind. We would witness as her belly grew, wishing so much that the baby was inside of me instead of her. Who was I kidding? I couldn't even stand being around close friends who were pregnant. How would I handle this? After the baby was born, if all went smoothly, we would have a beautiful addition to our family. But we mustn't forget the other addition to our family – there was a high likelihood that the birth mother would end up being a part of our lives forever. She might write to the child or have occasional visits or even take the child on outings. Our child might see her as the fun, younger mom that never disciplined and only did cool stuff. I had read that it was better for children to know their biological roots, and of course, I would do the right thing to ensure my child's optimal emotional wellbeing. But how would I handle maintaining a permanent "partnership" with this woman? Was I emotionally strong enough for this after everything that had happened?

    While taking a shower that evening - I do my best thinking in the shower - I thought further about all of the desperate couples like us who would be competing for years in the popularity contest to be matched with these prized babies. The more I thought about it, the more I realized that I would rather adopt a baby who didn't have hundreds of worthy couples competing for it. I would rather take a baby who might have some problems and needed a loving family as much as we needed a baby to care for. I was willing to risk having a child with disabilities. In any case of adoption, losing the baby after bonding with it was a huge fear. But if I were able to feel that I had given a child with rough beginnings a healthy dose of love and stability, it might lessen the pain of the loss somewhat.

After my shower, I sat down with James, and laid out my reasoning for wanting to go with a public adoption. I thought it would take some convincing, but to my amazement, he instantly agreed. He was excited about moving forward with building our family, and he was happy that we might be able to make a difference in the life of a disadvantaged child.

So the next day, I called the county and asked about what this process would entail. I discovered that we would have to take a class called "Pride" as well as a CPR class. We would do some paperwork and have our fingerprints taken. Next, we would get our house inspected and licensed as a foster home. At that point, we would be able to take in foster children. In order to adopt, we would also have to complete an adoption home study. This process consisted of more paperwork and a series of interviews. Once the home study was complete, we would be eligible to be matched with a child for adoption. The thought of being matched with a child started a parade of goosebumps up and down my arms. I wanted to get started right away, so I signed us up for the next available "Pride" class which would be starting on the coming Saturday.

Chapter 12
Pride

I didn't know what to expect from the "Pride" class, but I was pretty sure that if it was through the county, it wasn't likely to be an exceptionally worthwhile learning experience. I pictured something akin to traffic school, where you put in your time because you know you have to, but you don't really pull any useful information out of it.

The first day of class, James and I wandered in with about nine or ten other prospective foster parents. Two women stepped out in front of the class and introduced themselves as the instructors. Louanne, a jolly woman with long silver hair, was a foster mother who had successfully fostered at least 10 children. I was surprised to find out that the second teacher, Dina, was the child of two alcoholics, and had been removed from her biological parent's home at the age of 10. She had been raised by foster parents from that day forward. Far from being the broken person that one might expect her to be, Dina was a dynamic speaker with incredible poise and grace that drew me in from the moment I met her.

Dina and Louanne spent the first session discussing the nuts and bolts of the foster care system. They stressed that the central mandate of the system is to keep biological families together. While children are in foster care, most biological parents are given opportunities to reform their lives. They are required to complete certain steps such as taking parenting classes or going through drug rehabilitation, and the county provides them with the resources they need to accomplish these things. If the birth parents do all that is asked of them within a reasonable timeframe, they are reunited with their children. Even in the case of a foster-to-adopt placement, the goal is still to reunify with the biological parents. It is called "concurrent planning" - the fost-adopt parent must be there to support efforts at reunification but also is expected to be there to adopt if reunification fails. Even in a foster-to-adopt placement in which reunification fails, the process of adopting the child can vary depending on how much the biological parents fight. They can get appeal after appeal, sparking multiple continuances, dragging out the process literally for years.

The job of the foster parent is not an easy one. In addition to all of the barriers to adoption, foster parents are likely to have children with extremely challenging issues due to the neglect or abuse that led them to be removed from their biological families. Further, in our county, around 75% of the babies and children in the system were exposed in utero to drugs or alcohol, which can lead to varying degrees of physical, mental, educational, and emotional issues. I started to fidget in my seat as panic set in. This was much more daunting than I had pictured.

As if we were not already discouraged enough, our teachers next quoted the bleak statistics about the odds of getting a newborn baby that was completely free for adoption with no plan for reunification. This type of a placement only happens in very rare cases like when an infant is legally surrendered at a fire station or an Emergency Room. If we were to wait to be matched with a newborn baby who was free for adoption, it would most likely take many years.

Dina and Louanne, not wanting to send everyone in the room running for the hills, also stressed the significance of foster parents in the lives of the children. Louanne's foster children had been such difficult cases that prior foster parents were unable to handle them, and they had been bounced around from one home to another. Thanks to Louanne's patience and love for her children, they all stabilized and ended up becoming productive adults. Dina's life was saved by the foster family who took her in as a child, rescuing her from a family of alcoholism and violence. They taught her how to give and receive love and how to work toward her goals. They gave her unconditional love and stability that she had never known during the early, formative years of her life. And here she stood - an eloquent, accomplished woman who had earned a master's degree and had successfully raised two children of her own.

What an amazing difference foster parents could make in children's lives! It was just unfortunate that I clearly was not up for the challenge. As much as I wanted to help needy children, my fight or flight alarm bells were ringing, and I had no fight left in me. By the time the class was over, I was ready to bolt and never look back. I wanted to completely give up on the idea of adoption. It was clear that I was not strong enough to withstand the uncertainty and emotional vulnerability. This had been one of my worst ideas yet.

As James and I drove home, I turned to him ready to admit that my brainy idea had been a complete flop.

"What did you think?" I asked, giving him a chance to vent his frustration at the insurmountable obstacles thrown in front of our path to becoming new parents.

"I am so glad that you thought of this," he replied, smiling, "It seems like a great thing for us to do."

His response shocked me. I had been fully expecting his level of panic to be commensurate with mine.

"Really, you think we can actually do this?"

"Well, it does sound completely scary, but there are so many kids out there that need a good, stable home. When they were talking about those traumatized kids, I felt like they were describing me as a child."

James had never been removed from his home and placed in foster care, but he had experienced traumas over the course of his childhood. James' parents loved their children very much and worked hard to provide for them. But financial struggles and family conflicts dominated a large part of the landscape of James' youth. His father worked overseas and was absent for much of his childhood. When James was nine, his mother joined his father in the United States and left the five children behind in the Philippines under the care of relatives. The plan was for the parents to establish themselves in the States before sending for the children. At that young age, James couldn't comprehend what was happening or why his mother was abruptly absent. After about six months, James and his siblings joined their parents in the states. By that point, the marriage was in crisis. When James' father left for good, many adult responsibilities fell on the kids, and they all had to work like crazy just to keep the family afloat. I could see why James had such strong empathy for the children in the system. I could understand his desire to provide a child with an environment that allowed the innocence of childhood to flower over the dry weeds of the past.

I, on the other hand, had grown up in a very stable family where the only abuse that I ever suffered was inflicted by my own perfection-demanding brain. Yet here was James with strength enough for the both of us. His confidence settled my nerves. I realized that no path was going to be easy for us, so we might as well choose the path that does the most good for others. Once I resigned myself to the decision to move forward, I felt the excitement building again. I pictured the empty room in our house with a crib and a changing table and its new little occupant, peacefully sleeping.

The next few sessions of the Pride class were devoted to Positive Parenting. Dina took the lead on this topic. First she went through the brain development of a child and noted the parts of the brain that are under-developed with abused children. The brains of kids who have been drug-exposed or traumatized actually appear quite different when scanned. These children tend to function more in the lower portions of the brain where the fight or flight response is located. They become easily agitated and have a hard time accessing the limbic system of the brain which serves to soothe and calm. For these children especially, the only way to reach the thinking part of the brain is to get them calm. Dina proceeded to describe the ways in which we can create a calming environment for these children and move their functioning back, as much as possible, into the upper portions of their brains.

Dina cited numerous studies which have shown that children respond better to discipline that is focused on what they should do rather than what they shouldn't do. For example, it is more effective to say "walk on the sidewalk" rather than "don't go in the street" or "use gentle touch" rather than "no hitting." At first, this seemed like only a slightly different semantic that I wondered if kids were even sophisticated enough to detect. But the more Dina spoke, the more I could see that it made good sense. Being mindful of your words and constantly framing everything in a positive way trains your mind to think in a positive way about your child and about life in general. When consistently applied, it also sends the message to the child that you have positive feelings about him or her.

As we continued on with the remainder of the Pride class, James and I were amazed at how valuable this class would be for any parent, whether they were raising foster children or biological children. Dina provided us with specific strategies for countless different scenarios from how to get kids to clean their rooms to how to stand firm in negotiations with teenagers. I found myself using the techniques on Marsha, on coworkers, and even on myself! James and I both came out of the class invigorated. We were ready to deal with any challenge that any child could throw at us. Dina's positivity and energy was truly contagious. By the time we walked out of Pride class, we were looking at all aspects of life in a more positive way.

Chapter 13
XY

One morning, a month or so after my D&C, I got a call at work from Dr. Montana.

"Julie, the results of the chromosomal testing of the fetal tissue are back," Dr. Montana's voice was softer and less self-assured than normal. "The result was normal XY."

I was taken aback. I had fully expected the results to be normal, but I did not realize that I would find out the gender of the baby as well.

Dr. Montana continued, "The fact that the baby was a male makes us positive that we tested the baby's tissue and not yours. So this result tells us for sure that there was no chromosomal problem with the baby. I don't know what to tell you at this point. Since nothing turned up in the miscarriage battery, then you are in the dubious category of 'unexplained miscarriage'. You could keep trying, but the probability of success would go down with each failed attempt."

I thanked Dr. Montana, and we hung up. My mind flashed to the euphoric moment when James and I beheld our little baby's beating heart. The fact that he was a boy now made him more real to me. I sharply felt the intense emptiness of my womb. Our perfect baby boy had lived and died there. Every nerve in my body ached for him.

Now that I had gotten my answer that I had known all along, I was filled with more questions. I had to find out what was wrong with me that was making my uterus kill perfect babies. Dr. Montana had been a nice doctor, but my problems were clearly way out of his league. I figured there must be doctors out there who specialize in this type of problem.

XY

I did some research and found a reproductive endocrinologist at Stanford who specialized in recurrent miscarriage. As I stepped into her office, I was sure that she would be able to unravel the mystery that was turning my body into a walking cemetery. Dr. Locke was a tall slender woman with short blond hair who crinkled her nose when she smiled. She held my heavy chart in her lap, and proceeded to describe to me the four major causes of miscarriage.

"The first thing we suspect when someone miscarries is that it was a chromosomal abnormality. But the normal karyotype results of the two of you and this most recent fetus rule this out as the cause. The second possibility is that it is a hormonal problem, but that would have shown up on the blood tests which you took. Structural abnormalities of the uterus can also lead to recurrent miscarriage, but your hysteroscopy has ruled that out. The last category is thrombophilia, or the propensity of one's blood toward clotting. Your thrombophilia panel was normal, but that panel only looks at the most common causes of thrombophilia. There is no possible way to test for or even identify every conceivable cause of thrombophila." Dr. Locke looked up from my chart, "My guess is that you have thrombophilia. This causes tiny micro clots to form in the blood vessels of the placenta, which eventually disrupt the blood supply to the fetus. The good news is that this is a very treatable condition. We would put you on a blood thinner called Lovenox, which is administered by injection. It will not harm the baby, but it should keep your blood thin enough so that the micro clots do not form."

I had to suppress the urge to jump out of my seat and hug Dr. Locke! Finally here was someone who was willing to DO something to fix what was going wrong with me. Here was someone who did not want to blame my troubles on bad luck statistically tantamount to being struck by lightning indoors during a California summer. This theory made a lot of sense. I never bled very much no matter how badly I was cut. I also remembered that at the age of two, I developed a blood clot in my brain when I tumbled head-first off of my brother's bed. I must have blood that just loves to clot.

Eagerly, we signed up to take the Lovenox, and do another cycle with Clomid and intrauterine insemination. Two injections of Lovenox per day sounded a tad overwhelming, but I could probably get used to it. With such a high frequency of injections, I knew I had to stop leaning on James and get used to doing them on my own.

I soon realized that Lovenox was a whole different ballgame from the hcg shot that James had heroically administered several months back. The Lovenox needle was considerably thicker and actually took a good deal of force to penetrate the skin. The medicine itself wreaked havoc on all of the surrounding tissue, sending every nerve ending in the vicinity on a shooting rampage. No matter how slowly I plunged in the medicine, I couldn't escape the feeling that hundreds of bees were stinging my abdomen from the inside. It would sometimes throb for a good half-hour after the shot. And my pincushion belly was developing dark indigo leopard spots of bruises. I wouldn't be wearing any bikinis for a while! Each time I administered the shot, I tried to picture that I was giving my baby a pre-natal bottle of sorts, delivering what was needed to sustain life. This image got my hands to do what was necessary.

The first insemination did the trick, and by mid-October, I was pregnant for the fourth time. But this time would be different - the baby was now getting what it needed to keep the life-giving vessels flowing from the placenta. Our six and a half week ultrasound revealed a vigorously beating heart delivering the wonderfully clot-free blood to the baby's body. Even though this was a beautiful sight, I did not allow myself to relax at this point. In the previous pregnancy, we had seen the heart still beating at almost seven weeks. The next week's ultrasound would be the true test.

Even though I knew that this baby was getting the necessary medicine, I was resolved to not leave anything to chance. If we were to lose the baby, I didn't want anything delayed in terms of our adoption. So James and I continued with wrapping up the licensing and home study process. We got fingerprinted and TB tested, took a CPR class, filled out stacks of paperwork for the adoption home study, and did our preliminary interviews with the home study worker. Although all of the people we came in contact with throughout this process were very nice, the process itself was quite intrusive. We were asked in-depth questions about our motivations, our parenting philosophies, and the state of our marriage. One question even asked us to write in detail about the last argument that James and I had and how we resolved the issue! It felt so wrong that I should be inspected in such granular detail in order to become a parent, when criminals and drug-addicts could repeatedly earn the title at will. Yet I understood that if the county was going to place innocent children in the care of adoptive parents, they had an obligation to be as thorough as possible in order to ensure that the prospective parents were fit and prepared.

Chapter 14
Signs From On High

On the night before our seven and a half week ultrasound, the short intervals during which I slept were haunted by nightmares. I helplessly watched as puppies fell off bridges, armed gunmen randomly shot hostages, and I showed up late to various teaching jobs, unprepared and unable to find the classroom. I woke up battle-worn and dreading the terrifying images the day might have in store for me. I prayed that the Lovenox shots had been doing their job to change the course of our recurring nightmare. As we took the ramp onto I-280, I felt like we were on our way to face a firing squad. We had done this so many times now that there really wasn't much to say. We just each sat in our own separate cocoons, bracing ourselves for what we would have to deal with in the coming hour. Glancing out in the direction of Stanford, I spotted a rainbow peacefully hanging over our destination. I pointed it out to James, and we stared at it together, both praying that it was some kind of divine sign, gently summoning us to our own personal pot of gold.

Lately, we had seen so many things that could only be interpreted as signs from God. A few weeks before, as we sat in a restaurant, James pointed out a beautiful boy about six years old, with brown hair and almond eyes. James commented that the boy looked a lot like our imagined son might look. As we were longingly gazing at him, his father called from the table, "Isaac, come back here please!" James and I both got chills. That was supposed to be our son's name. Could this be a sign that our Isaac was on his way?

James and I had recently visited a home in the foothills of Redwood City to take a look at a car that was for sale. The woman who answered the door was a plain woman, with gray hair pulled back in a bun. She looked to be in her late forties – a bit young to have a full head of gray hair. She smiled warmly and invited us into her home. We sat down with her for a bit and listened as she spoke lovingly of her grown son and daughter who had both moved away. Her son had set her up with a computer and Internet access so that they could still keep in touch on a daily basis. Despite the continuous contact with her children, she still seemed lonely. Attempting to lengthen our visit, she showed us around the downstairs of her house, pointing out the various works of art she had created in the pottery class which she took to pass the time. We didn't mind the lengthy stay because we really enjoyed her company and her simple, sweet manner. When James went out with her to test drive the car, they spoke further, and it somehow came up in the conversation that we were having recurrent miscarriages. She confided in James that her first three pregnancies had also ended in miscarriages. She was desperate to start a family and felt completely hopeless because her husband refused to consider adoption. So she kept trying, and miraculously, her fourth and fifth pregnancies produced two perfectly healthy children.

    Not only did we like this woman, but we also liked the car she was selling, which we bought at a very reasonable price. When we returned home, James told me what she had revealed to him during their drive. I felt a huge wave of relief as I realized for the first time that I was not completely alone in the world. There was someone else who actually understood what I was going through. This woman must have been as drawn to us as we were to her because we shared an invisible bond that very few people share. We had been through the exact same heartbreak, decades apart. I felt that she must have been some sort of a messenger from God, delivering us hope that our story would end like hers, with children who would live and grow, and cause us to miss them terribly when they left home.

    My mind reviewed all of these divine signs as I waited for Dr. Locke to illuminate the secret world of my uterus. I clung to them like a security blanket, and they wrapped themselves around me, keeping the monsters at bay. Dr. Locke located the baby quickly, and I immediately saw on the ultrasound screen the products of the good work of Lovenox. There in a perfectly round gestational sac was a 7 ½ week old baby with a fully functional heart!

"Everything looks great," Dr. Locke said.

"Really," I replied, my voice shaky, "Are you sure?"

"Yes," my good doctor confidently responded, "This is exactly how things should look at this stage. We'll see you back next week, and continue monitoring you until ten weeks. Then your regular OB can take over."

With that, Dr. Locke ripped the printed images off of the ultrasound and handed one to me. I couldn't believe what I had in my hand. We had made it to the major milestone that most couples take for granted at their very first ultrasound. We were taking home a picture of our child! At all of our other ultrasounds, the doctors would quietly tuck the ultrasound images away into my chart because either the baby had been dead or it was so early that they didn't want to give us a photographic remembrance for a pregnancy that still was quite iffy. But here it was in my hands, and I could look at my baby now any time I wanted to.

As soon as Dr. Locke closed the door, James and I held each other tightly and sobbed. Holding him was the only thing that was keeping my entire body from shaking as the stress leading up to this moment was set free in one giant tsunami.

My 8 ½ week ultrasound appointment occurred the week of Thanksgiving of 2005. I fidgeted as I sat on the exam table waiting for Dr. Locke to arrive to do the scan.

"I wonder if I'll ever be able to relax for one of these," I said to James as my fingers aimlessly poked a hole in the paper sheet that covered my legs.

"I know," James responded, "I wonder how many years all this stress has taken off of our life spans."

The Lovenox had made me feel much better about things intellectually, but in my heart, I was still just as uneasy as ever.

Signs From On High

"Doctors always have to run late for ultrasound appointments, don't they?" I vented.

James grabbed a magazine and tried to pass the time leafing through it with me. The choice of magazines at Stanford REI was quite humble. Luckily the Stanford staff was sensitive enough to not fill the room with pregnancy and parenting magazines. However, the term boring was a generous description for what they did offer – mostly golf and real estate magazines. Knowing nothing about golf, we opted to leaf through a publication which featured the homes for sale in Alameda County.

After we had viewed what seemed like every home in the county, Dr. Locke rushed in, apologizing for the delay. She got right down to business and started the ultrasound. She located the sac, and proceeded to press buttons and re-orient the wand.

"Well I see quite a bit of growth from last week." Dr. Locke sounded encouraged.

My breathing became shallow and rushed, "Is there a heartbeat?" I asked pleadingly.

"I don't have a good view of it," she replied as she pushed more buttons and fiddled with the wand. More silence. More fiddling. Then she finally spoke.

"I don't see a heartbeat," Dr. Locke looked up at me. "I'm sorry Julie."

My mind reeled in disbelief. There was no way that this could be happening to us again. The Lovenox was supposed to be the answer.

"Does this mean that clotting wasn't the problem after all? Or was the dosage of Lovenox not high enough?" I asked, desperate to hear that there was some sort of explanation.

"We can't know for sure." Dr. Locke responded, "It could be that this one had a chromosomal abnormality. Just because the last one was chromosomally normal doesn't mean that this one was."

The fact that she was falling back on the old standby, the chromosomal abnormality, meant that she had absolutely no idea what was going on. This wasn't a chromosomal abnormality. This was the same demon that had silently drained the lives of my other three children. We knew it, and she knew it. The expert in recurrent miscarriages was clueless when it came to my pathetic excuse for a body.

As James and I unsteadily walked out of the clinic, it hit me how low the odds were that we would ever have a biological child. Thus far, I had always thought that it would happen, and it was just a matter of time and patience. But at this point I realized that if even the top expert at Stanford was mystified, there may be nothing that anyone could do to make this happen. As I stepped outside, I felt like an invisible bubble surrounded me, separating me from the rest of the reproducing world. The other women on the street walked with the confidence that they could experience life's quintessential experience. They could create life and count on their bodies to nurture it. They could bring that precious life into the world and sustain it at their breast. They could give children to their husbands, grandchildren to their parents, nieces and nephews to their siblings. They were not defective in the most fundamental way as I was.

I wondered why James wanted to stay with me. My body had been responsible for the theft of our newlywed bliss. My body had sabotaged his chance to continue his blood line, to nurture a part of himself and see his legacy continue with his grandchildren and great-grandchildren. He could easily leave me and find someone who could give him that gift. I imagined that his family must wish that he had chosen another woman, one who could bear children for him. They definitely never expressed anything but love for me, but who could possibly want this kind of a life for their loved-one? I had brought nothing but pain and suffering into his life and theirs in turn. Everyone, including myself, would be better off if I just didn't exist.

Dr. Locke performed the D&C the next day, and I fought against the nurse trying to wake me up from the procedure. If only there was some way that I could remain in the shelter of the anesthesia-induced coma forever. In my dreams, I could be someone else. I could experience the relief of temporary amnesia. Each time I woke up, I would be forced to remember why my head was pounding, my nose was stuffed, and my eyes were sore and swollen. Waking up continually triggered me to relive the instant that the bad news was delivered, and my dreams vanished into thin air.

The day after the D&C was Thanksgiving Day. We sent Marsha off with my parents to visit my dad's family. James and I weren't feeling very social or very thankful. We stayed in bed most of the day and drifted in and out of sleep, sobbing off and on and just holding each other. What was there to be thankful for? I deeply loved James and Marsha and the rest of my family, but at this moment, I was not thankful that they were in my life. They deserved someone better than me. Not only was I unable to bear a child, but I was doing a pathetic job with the one I already had. My obsession with reproduction had stolen my focus from Marsha more than any actual baby ever could have. I was depressed and distant half the time. My mind was always busily processing my grief or methodically planning the next steps, and there was little room left for anything else. At this point, I could think of nothing in my life that I hadn't royally screwed up.

And where was God in all of this? Had all of the signs that James and I had seen along the way in this pregnancy been some sort of cruel joke from God - building us up as much as possible before dropping the bomb? More likely, they had not been signs at all. Our minds were so desperate for relief that we just saw whatever we wanted to see. Coincidences became divine intervention. Sometimes, perhaps all the time, a rainbow is just a rainbow.

Chapter 15
A Sister of a Friend of a Cousin

Upon recovering from the D&C number four, I placed all of my energy into completing the final requirements for our foster adoption. By this time, the licensing home visit was less than a week away, and our house still had a long way to go to comply with the lengthy list of requirements. Mercifully distracted from our grief, James and I worked tirelessly. We locked up the medicines, cleaners, and knives, tested the smoke detectors, covered the electrical outlets, and scoured every inch in between. James assembled a crib in our spare bedroom to be ready at a moment's notice for a tiny tenant.

One afternoon as I was inspecting the house against the checklist, the phone rang. It was a pleasant surprise to hear from my cousin Paul. Only two months apart in age and one town apart in family homes, Paul and I had grown up side by side, sharing countless adventures. As adults now with separate, busy lives, our contact with each other was much less frequent, but I always felt Paul's support and sincere sympathy for what James and I were going through.

"Hey Paul, how are you doing?" I replied.

"I'm good. Hey listen, I heard that you and James are thinking about adopting a baby. My friend Bill's sister, Kelsey is looking for an adoptive home for her eight week old baby girl, and I was thinking that you guys might be interested."

The checklist fell from my hands, and I dropped into the nearest chair. "Um, we might be interested. Can you tell me more? Why is she giving up an eight week old baby?"

"Well it seems that she gave the baby up for adoption at birth, but she had some problems with the adoptive parents.

I don't know all the details, but it sounds like they had agreed to keep in contact with her and send her pictures, but after the baby was born, they refused. So she ended up taking the baby back. But she still wants to put her up for adoption, and wants to find another adoptive couple as soon as possible."

A tornado of red flags whipped around my body. Getting involved with this girl, who had already reneged on one adoptive couple, seemed like an ill-advised move. Still, I couldn't ignore this opportunity which had just fallen into my lap. The thought of having a tiny baby girl in such near term was impossible to resist. The skin on my arms warmed as I imagined them wrapped around a peacefully nestled infant.

"What do you know about Kelsey?" I asked Paul. "Do you think we can trust her?"

"I don't know too much about her, to be honest. My impression from Bill is that she is immature, but I'm pretty sure she's not into any serious trouble like drugs or anything." Paul responded.

I told Paul that I would get back to him. When I laid out the story for James, an expression of panic emerged across his face. He was also unsure whether Providence was swooping in with a heavenly-stamped care package or winding up to deliver the knock-out punch.

I thought back on what I knew about Kelsey's family. Many years ago, Bill had been seriously ill, and my aunt had cared for Kelsey and her younger brother for a long period of time while their mother stayed with Bill in the hospital. I recalled my aunt being amazed by how intelligent and sweet the kids were (good genes for the baby to inherit!). Bill's mom was unable to run her business while taking care of her sick son, and the family struggled to make ends meet. At the time, as a teenager, my heart went out to them, so I anonymously donated a couple hundred dollars to help out. The thought crossed my mind that somehow the good karma from our family helping their family may be coming back around to us. Maybe it was somehow predestined that our families should be cosmically linked.

All mystical prophesies aside, I knew for sure that the opportunity to take home an infant girl who came from a nice family and was not exposed to drugs and alcohol was not something that came around every day. And the chance to have this baby right now instead of potentially waiting for years made my heart give in and take the plunge. Next thing I knew, I was wading past all of the red flags and fixing my radar on the new goal at hand. This baby was meant for us, and I was going to see to it the events played out as fate intended.

Of course, if this was something that was written in the stars, then fate theoretically shouldn't need my help to make it happen. Nevertheless, I was committed. I pitched to James all the reasons that this was a great idea, and downplayed all of the potential risks. He agreed that we should at least find out more details, so I let Paul know that we were interested in finding out more and would like Kelsey to contact us.

The next day, as I was driving home from work, my cell phone rang. A monotonic voice responded to my greeting.

"Hi, this is Kelsey Williams." She paused. "My brother Bill gave me your number. He said you were interested in the baby."

I took a deep breath. *Stay calm. Think carefully before you speak.*

"Hi Kelsey. Thanks so much for calling." I responded, "Yes, we are very interested in the baby. We would love to meet you and get more information."

That evening, Kelsey's tentative knock on our door sent both our hearts into an arrhythmic shudder. Closing the dogs in the family room, James and I went for the front door. As both dogs barked and obnoxiously hurled themselves against the glass door, I began to panic. What if she didn't like dogs? What if she didn't like the house? What if she couldn't stand me?

James swung open the door, and we took our first look at half the genes of our potential daughter. Kelsey was beautiful - tall and slender, with long auburn hair. Her face resembled a tired and slightly sullen version of Jennifer

Garner. Her mad-at-the-world expression gave my stomach a jab of dread. How awkward and painful was this encounter going to be?

We invited her in and introduced ourselves. Kelsey's eyes widened as she noticed our dogs.

"You have dogs!" Kelsey exclaimed. "I love dogs! Can they come out and play?"

"Of course," James smiled, "As long as you don't mind getting licked to death."

I slid open the glass door, and two happy flashes of fur bounded over to our visitor. Kelsey had been true to her word that she didn't mind their eager tongues, as she stooped down on the floor and played with them, freely accepting their affection.

I felt instant relief that we had so quickly found a point of connection with Kelsey in our mutual love of dogs. James showed off the tricks that Nigel and Winnie could do. I beamed with pride at our impressive little pair as they performed synchronized sitting, spinning, and rolling. We sat and played with the dogs for a while and Kelsey talked a lot about her dog. It turned out that Kelsey worked part time at a pet store, and her dream was to become a dog groomer.

Eventually, we moved the conversation to the kitchen. I offered Kelsey some dinner, and she eagerly ate and sipped tea. Fiddling with her tea bag, she tearfully told the story of the one-night stand at a party that led to her pregnancy. Soon after that fateful night, she met and started dating her current boyfriend. When she found out she was pregnant, she was devastated. She didn't want her parents or her boyfriend to find out, so she made an appointment at an abortion clinic. The day of the appointment, she decided that she couldn't go through with it. She didn't want to raise the baby, but she also didn't want to end its life. So she courageously opted to put the baby up for adoption which forced her to confess to everyone. I was amazed by the maturity of this decision. I was getting more and more comfortable with Kelsey being my baby's birth mom.

To her surprise, her parents and her boyfriend were supportive of her. She searched for an adoptive couple and found one that she got along with well. As she progressed through the pregnancy, her boyfriend stood by her and they both mourned the loss the day that the baby girl was born and handed over to the adoptive couple.

Once they had the child, the adoptive parents suddenly turned on Kelsey. They had agreed to update her on how the baby was doing and to send her pictures from time to time. But after the baby was born, they cut off all communication with Kelsey. When Kelsey forced the issue, and the adoptive mother grudgingly spoke to her, she sounded disgusted with Kelsey and overwhelmed with the baby. Kelsey decided that this arrangement wasn't going to work. She hadn't asked the couple for much. She didn't ask to be involved in the baby's life. She simply wanted some updates so that she could be reassured that the baby was doing well. When Kelsey told them that she had changed her mind and wanted to find a different adoptive couple, they agreed with very little resistance. Obviously this was a really bad match for all involved.

Since then, Kelsey's mother had been caring for the baby, but she had no intention of raising her. Worried that she would get overly attached to her granddaughter, she had urged Kelsey to find a new adoptive home as quickly as possible.

As Kelsey ran through the Kleenex box we had placed in front of her, I really felt for her. How devastating it must be to have to give up a baby not once, but twice. I admired her strength and was beginning to really like her. I sensed that she was feeling the same about us.

We got along a little too well, in fact. Kelsey stayed at our house and poured her heart out about her childhood, her boyfriend, her dog, her plans for the future, and every topic in between. Even though I was comfortable with her, I was still completely nervous about the entire encounter. I felt that we had to say and do everything perfectly right in order to keep her impressed with us. By 11:00, I was completely exhausted from being in self-monitoring overdrive for so long.

Kelsey agreed to bring the baby the following day so that we could meet her. I was delighted that things were progressing so well. But I was petrified to meet the baby. What if she cried when I held her? What if I was so nervous that I wouldn't be able to put her at ease? I had been purposely avoiding infants for the past few years because they made me feel so sad. Would I remember how to calm her, feed her, burp her? Would Kelsey think that I wouldn't be a fit mother? It was extremely exhausting to have to audition for motherhood.

The following day was a Saturday, and early in the morning, the phone rang. I answered it, and heard a cheerful voice on the other end.

"Hi, this is Janet Williams, Kelsey's mother."

"Oh hi," I reciprocated her cheery tone, jumping back into high self-monitoring mode, "It's great to hear from you. How are you doing?"

"I'm so excited that you guys might get the baby! Kelsey is only looking at one other couple, and they are in Sacramento. If the baby went there, we'd probably never see her."

Now I understood the excitement in her tone. Janet wanted to be the grandma even though Kelsey wasn't going to be the mother. It was not a surprise that she felt that way, especially since she was caring for the baby now. In my view, it's not possible for a kid to have too many grandparents. Marsha, besides my parents, my grandparents, and James' parents, has two sets of biological grandparents with whom she keeps in touch. One is local and sees her quite frequently. It has never been a problem. In fact, it has always been a benefit for her to have a positive link to her biological side. So I reassured Janet that we sincerely welcomed her involvement if we were to raise the baby. Janet was elated. She arranged to bring the baby in a couple of hours. The staccato pulse of my heart echoed in my ears as my brain wrestled with the weight of what was about to happen. I couldn't believe we were about to meet this little person who might actually become our daughter!

As promised, a couple of hours later, we heard a knock at the door. We eagerly opened the door, and there stood Kelsey, her mother and her father. I wasn't expecting the whole family! But I quickly ignored that thought as my focus zeroed in on the infant seat hanging off of Janet's hand. That was her! She was in there!

We ushered the family in. Kelsey quietly went to the back room to see Marsha. It was clear she didn't want to be near the baby. I on the other hand was dying to catch my first glimpse. As Janet placed the seat on the floor and removed the heavy blankets, I was finally able to peer in at the peacefully sleeping girl. She was exquisite. Her soft, auburn hair settled perfectly on her porcelain forehead like it had been professionally cut. The pacifier in her tiny mouth was gently bobbing up and down, slightly rocking her pink, pinchable cheeks. Her elegant, slender hands rested on the front of her purple dress, gently swaying with each breath. A hand-crafted doll could never be made to match the beauty of this little girl. A being so extraordinary could only be referred to as baby with a capital B.

"She is so beautiful!" I exclaimed.

"Would you like to hold her?" Janet asked, beaming with pride.

"Well, I don't want to disturb her." I said, holding back my strong desire to whisk her up and never let go.

"She'll be waking up soon anyway." Janet smiled, and started to unlatch her straps.

I took a deep breath. How was it going to feel to hold her for the first time? Would I feel an instant connection that would let me know that this was my daughter as opposed to just a fantastically beautiful baby? Janet tenderly lowered her into my arms. She felt soft and warm. Still asleep, her relaxed body form-fitted to the cradle of my arms. She breathed deeply and peacefully, unaware of the significance of the moment.

Janet smiled. "She looks right at home in your arms."

I could scarcely believe that this was happening. Less than a month ago, my fourth baby was being vacuumed out of my body, and here I was holding a baby that could be mine within days!

Slight squirming interrupted my reverie. Still focused on Baby's face, I watched as a pair of brilliant, blue eyes were slowly unveiled. The drowsy girl squinted for a few moments and then committed to a wakeful state. As she surveyed the room, I remarked at how alert she was for such a young baby. I was sure that she was going to be as bright as she was beautiful.

Baby remained relaxed as Janet reviewed with me her basic routine. James sat beside me and made faces at the attentive girl. Her eyes lit up and her mouth rounded into an awkward smile as she watched her goofy prospective daddy.

"Would you like to hold her?" I asked James, realizing that I was completely monopolizing the precious girl.

James reached out his arms to Baby, and drew her close to his chest. His eyes welled up as he breathed her in. For a time, James, Baby, and I were the only people in the world. We exchanged silly faces, made babble small talk, and gazed at each other in happily acquainted amazement. After an hour or two, Janet indicated that they needed to get going. As Grandma, Grandpa, and Baby departed, Kelsey remained. I wished that a different set of three people would have left, but I realized that we did need to finalize things with Kelsey.

Again, Kelsey stayed and stayed, telling us more stories of her life. I was very interested in learning all there was to know about her, but wished that it didn't have to be done all at once. The emotions of the day had drained my energy entirely. I worried that if this went on much longer, I would be dozing off to Kelsey's life drama which would certainly tarnish her impression of me. I straightened my sitting position in an effort to remain attentive.

At some point, Kelsey said the words I was waiting to hear. "Ok, I'm comfortable with this," she said, "I will have my mom bring the baby tomorrow, and then we can work out the paperwork later."

My urge to sleep transformed into an urge to dance and shout. James and I hugged Kelsey and told her how grateful we were to her that she had chosen us. We reassured her that we would do the best job we possibly could in raising the baby. We told her how much we respected and admired her for protecting the baby's life and taking care in selecting an adoptive home. Kelsey seemed like she wanted to say more, but she smiled and headed for the door.

And with that, she was gone. James and I collapsed into each other's arms and didn't let go. Our bad luck had finally ended! Our baby girl would be home tomorrow. The hugeness of this concept could not be contained in my perception. We sat down together and soaked in the moment. I looked down at my arms which still radiated with the sensation of cozy baby. A montage of crackly reel-to-reel footage spooled through my brain. A crimson-haired girl with a mischievous smile took her first wobbly steps, raced her bicycle down a tree-lined street, and lofted her graduation cap into the air.

Within a couple of hours after calling our family to tell them the amazing news, my mother and grandmother arrived at the door with a flood of cards, gifts, and hand-me-downs from various family members. Tears wildly streaked down my face as I unpacked the tiny things that my daughter would soon be wearing. Late that evening, we finally finished getting everything put away and ready for Baby.

The next morning, we anxiously awaited Janet's call. Around 11:00, the caller id popped up with her number. I quickly scooped up the phone.

"Hi Janet," I said cheerfully.

"Hi Julie," The voice on the other end lacked the lilt of exuberance that had been present the other day. Suddenly I flashed back to the exam table, waiting for the doctor to break the silence and tell me what had become of my baby. "Kelsey would like to talk with you one more time before bringing the baby."

"What's going on? Is there a problem?" I responded. I saw the look on the doctor's face. I saw the motionless sac.

"Well, I don't think so," Janet was working hard to sound reassuring. "Kelsey can be so immature sometimes. She has been wanting to bring up money, and can't seem to find an opportunity. She has some medical expenses that need to be paid. That was part of the agreement with the previous couple – another part that they refused to follow through with."

"Ok," I replied, "When would she like to come over?"

"How about in an hour or so," Janet replied, "I'm sure you guys can work this out."

"Ok," I agreed, "We'll be here."

The doctor in my mind struggled to visualize the figure floating in the sac. This situation would require another scan, another session of excruciating limbo. Another soul crushing walk on the fine line separating ecstasy and devastation.

I went back over what Janet had said. I wondered what amount of money we were talking about. Since James and I had just bought a house, we didn't have sacks of cash lying around. I had researched the money involved in doing a private adoption. The home study alone would be around $8000. And then there would be lawyers to pay to handle the actual adoption, which was probably also around $8000. Plus, my plan had been to quit work when the baby came.

But the more I thought about it, I couldn't imagine that medical expenses could add up to that much. MediCal should have fully covered prenatal care and the birth. Maybe there were some copayments or vitamins or something. Or maybe she had some special tests done that were requested by the other adoptive family and weren't covered. The total must be somewhere around $1000. It had to be high enough for Kelsey to be afraid to bring it up, but I couldn't think of any medical expenses that could make it much higher than that. It was a routine, easy pregnancy.

So James and I figured we'd make it as easy as possible for Kelsey. We wrote up an agreement saying that should the baby be placed with us, we would agree to pay __ amount to cover the medical expenses of Kelsey Williams. We figured she could fill in the blank, and we could breeze past the awkwardness.

When Kelsey arrived, we presented her with the paper. She had a pained expression on her face.

"I had it all totaled up for the other couple. It wasn't just medical expenses. It was other things like maternity clothes, my rent." She paused and cast her eyes to the floor. "It all came out to around $20,000."

James and I sat in stunned silence.

"I have to tell you Kelsey," James stated, "That's a lot more than we were expecting."

Kelsey burst into tears. "I wouldn't ask for it if I didn't really need it. I am $10,000 in debt, and I need another $10,000 to pay for dog grooming school. I'm paying rent now for both myself and the baby at my parents' house. I just don't know what to do."

I could not believe what I was hearing. These expenses were not pregnancy related. Kelsey was selling the baby to get out of financial trouble. How could she get us hooked and then drop a bomb like this? I wanted a chance to talk with James about what we should do, but Kelsey was sitting there, waiting for a response from us.

"Kelsey," I said. "We are a young couple. We just bought a house. We don't have money like that lying around."

Kelsey didn't respond. She looked at the floor and sniffled. The temperature of my face was on the rise. My heart was racing. I felt Baby slipping away. I had to think of something to do to hold on to her. We couldn't give Kelsey $20,000 and pay for the adoption fees and then have money to raise a kid with. Besides that, I wouldn't feel right about paying for a baby. Was that even legal? There must be some way to frame this so that we could keep the baby and not go broke and not feel completely dirty. I thought about Kelsey's debt. I didn't feel right exchanging a baby for debt relief, but there were things I could do to help her with it. I could help her to manage it and get low interest rates. I could even help her file for bankruptcy if that was what the situation required. She was so young. By the time the seven year wait period to clear up her credit was over, she'd only be 26. I could even see paying her dog grooming school tuition as a gesture. After all, we wanted our baby's birth mother to be successful. We could scrape up the money somehow. We'd sell one of our cars if necessary.

I proposed the idea to James and Kelsey. Everyone seemed satisfied. She promised to bring the baby for real tomorrow, and promptly left. I had a sick feeling in the pit of my stomach. Though Baby was still within reach, I felt like I needed to take ten showers to wash off the scum of that transaction. No matter how I couched the terms, we were buying a baby. It was wrong, but I was that desperate. Also, we were losing our trust in Kelsey. What would prevent her from bringing the baby and then coming back and demanding more money? Was that what really happened with the other couple?

The next day, James and I moved about the house quietly. We avoided the nursery, which was now full of everything but a baby. At about midday, Kelsey called. James answered the phone. He listened for a moment and then covered up the mouthpiece and whispered to me.

"She said that she's looked into filing bankruptcy and doesn't think it will be as easy as we described. She wants to give us the baby, but the other couple is willing to pay the full $20,000."

I collapsed and started sobbing. James handled the conversation with Kelsey. He told her that she had now broken an agreement with us twice, and we had lost all trust in her. I shuddered as the nails were driven into the coffin of yet another dream. It was officially over.

When James put the phone down, I completely lost it and started screaming uncontrollably. I don't remember what I said. Just primal ranting about how much I hated this life. James tried to calm me, but I was inconsolable. I didn't know what to do. Why were we so cursed?

James took my hands and spoke firmly to me, "We will get through this. We've gotten through worse." He held my face, and looked straight into my red and running eyes. "This was just a temporary distraction from our overall goal to do a foster adoption. We will move on with that, and we will be OK. Let's get away for a while. We'll go on a cruise with Marsha."

How could we ever be OK after this? This situation had seemed so perfect. But yet again, I was seeing signs from God that simply didn't exist. Where the hell was He? What kind of screwed up plan was this? That perfect, beautiful baby was about to be sold, and we were left with a thing-filled, infant-empty nursery. I sobbed in James' arms until I was lightheaded and dizzy, too tired to cry any more. Then we just sat in sick, empty silence.

Later in the day, my aunt called Janet and tried to get her to talk sense into Kelsey, even though James and I knew it was too late. Janet confirmed what I suspected that she was never charging Kelsey or the baby any rent. When I thought about it, $10,000 sounded steep for dog-grooming school as well. Pure and simple, Kelsey was just a con artist, preying on the most vulnerable people possible. I was completely disgusted that people like this were granted the grace to procreate, and I was not.

Luckily, I had been wise enough not to cancel our home inspection for the foster license which was actually scheduled to take place the following day. Our house was ready, but we were half-dead. We had to find the strength from somewhere. We needed to go through with it, if not just to keep that selfish baby-seller from having any power to deter us from our original plan.

I spent the morning of the inspection day with a cold compress on my face, trying to reduce the swelling. I stared at myself in the mirror as I applied makeup to cover as much as possible the fallout from yesterday's explosion. I was 29 years old, but the grief of the past few years had carved irreversible lines on my face. My hair was going gray faster than I could pluck the wiry rascals. Something had to change soon.

Our home inspection went amazingly smoothly. Ruben, our licensing worker, was kind and friendly. He put us at ease, and temporarily took our minds off of the disaster from the day before. Satisfied with the state of our house, he congratulated us, informing us that we were officially a foster family home. I knew that this was the right path for us. We would not build our family by participating in a filthy abandonment of moral values. Our home would be a refuge for another soul who knew the unfair suffering that was randomly dealt out in this world. We would descend into the darkness of that baby's world and together rise up, so strong that nothing would ever bring us down again.

Chapter 16
Larger than Life

A couple of weeks after Hurricane Kelsey, we left on that cruise that James had aptly suggested. It was the inexpensive standard starter cruise - a four day jaunt to Catalina Island and Ensenada, Mexico. Having never been on a cruise, we didn't know what to expect. We just knew that we needed a change of scenery.

In what had become the hallmark of Aguas luck, Marsha came down with the flu the very day we left for the cruise. She still wanted to come, so we loaded her up on Tylenol and took her along, hoping that she would make a quick recovery. What a trooper she was taking the long flight and waiting in the lines to board the ship with a temperature of 102! She didn't complain one bit. As we pulled down her bed in our small cabin, she was so relieved to curl up and sleep.

By dinner-time, she had slept through the afternoon and was feeling a bit better, so she came to the dining room with us. Upon arriving at our assigned table, I discovered with disappointment that we were going to be seated with another family. I was not feeling particularly social, and wanted to just remain isolated within our own little battered family unit.

As we sat and perused the menu, a well-dressed woman in her mid-to-late 40s arrived at our table with two blond boys. She appeared to be very well-off with processed hair and freshly manicured hands. I didn't feel like I would have much in common with this woman. But since we'd be stuck with her for better or worse for all of our meals, we stood up smiling, and introduced ourselves. Her smile softened her appearance. I got the impression that she smiled a lot.

"Hi, I'm Olena, and these are my sons Sasha and John." Olena spoke with a thick Russian accent as she warmly outstretched her hand. As we shook hands and introduced our family, I felt a connection with Olena that I didn't expect. It just felt good to be with her. Her two little boys were polite and friendly. Sasha was 12 years old. He spoke with an adorable little trace of a Russian accent. A strikingly handsome boy, he had a mischievous grin accented by a pair of endearing dimples. Though he was a tiny boy for a 12 year old, he carried himself with the poise of someone much older and much taller. John was six years old, and was almost as tall as Sasha. He smiled sweetly as he interacted with us, frequently snuggling his cheek against Olena's sleeve.

Sasha and Marsha got along well right away. They chatted throughout dinner, comparing video games and favorite TV programs. James, Olena, and I also really clicked. Far from the pampered socialite that I mistook her for initially, she was actually a cardiologist. She had traveled the world, and had a lot of stories and insight. I was drawn to her unassuming and loving manner. I could tell by the way she looked at her children that being a mother was the most important thing in the world to her. She beamed with pride and love each time she looked at or spoke of her children. I could understand why. They were both wonderful little boys. Sasha especially was so magnetic and charming that I could not help smiling whenever he was around.

After a couple of meals with them, we ventured out together to other parts of the ship, taking the kids to the karaoke bar. Sasha was so excited about having a turn at karaoke. Marsha wanted to try it, but was reluctant to get up in front of everyone. Sasha encouraged Marsha.

"Come on. It'll be so much fun. It doesn't matter how you sound." He convinced her, and the two walked over to put their names on the list. While they were gone, Olena and I sat smiling.

"Sasha is absolutely enchanting," I said to Olena.

"Thank you Sweetheart." Olena responded. "He has come a long way."

I was puzzled, wondering what he had come a long way from.

Olena continued, "I adopted Sasha from Russia. He was the child of an alcoholic mother, who left him with his father when he was a baby. When he was seven years old, his father abandoned him as well, leaving him in a busy train station. I adopted him from a Russian orphanage when he was ten years old."

I couldn't believe what I was hearing. Sasha was so well adjusted. How could it be that two years ago, he was living in a Russian orphanage, abandoned by both his parents? How could not one but two parents abandon that beautiful child?

"You have done an incredible job with him," I told Olena, "He is such a sweet and confident boy. I would never have guessed what he has been through."

"He had a lot to overcome when he first came to us," Olena responded, "At first, he was very wild and angry. He lied all the time. It took some time for him to settle down."

"I'm so glad that you were there for him," I said to Olena, "I hate to imagine that amazing boy growing up in an orphanage."

At that moment, the DJ announced Sasha's name and he joyfully skipped onto the stage clutching the microphone. He belted out the most enthusiastic rendition ever to be heard of "Larger than Life" by the Backstreet Boys. He didn't hit a single note on key, but it didn't matter. The crowd was on its feet cheering for him. Despite his diminutive size and his unfortunate circumstances, this boy was truly larger than life. Everyone in the room was energized by the way he communicated the sheer joy of life.

The next name announced belonged to my beautiful daughter Marsha. She walked on stage with grace and poise that surprised me. I was worried that she would be too nervous singing in front of such a large crowd. She still had some cold symptoms from her lingering illness too. But as she sang the first few lines of Sarah Mclachlan's "Fallen," all of my fears vanished. She sang like I'd never heard her sing before. And she, unlike Sasha, did hit the notes right on. James and Olena and I joined the crowd in wild cheering and applause. What tremendous children these two were! Both had extraordinarily traumatic starts in life, and both were making the world a more beautiful place for everyone they encountered.

    I shared Marsha's adoption story with Olena at a later time. Our similar experiences must be what made us such kindred spirits from the get-go. When we finished the cruise, we sadly parted ways with our dining companions, exchanging email addresses and vowing to keep in touch. Both James and I came home from the cruise rejuvenated and filled with eager anticipation of the next chapter in our adoption story.

Chapter 17
A Day Like Any Other

When you wake up in the morning on a day that changes your life, there is no hint of what is to come. On Thursday, January 5, 2006, I woke up with the same dull ache that accompanied every morning. Just as it was the day before, I pleaded with my alarm clock to prolong the snooze just a little bit and let me remain in the world of my dreams. When the alarm clock denied my request as it always did, I was dragged back into my unfriendly reality. I heard the same painful echo of the souls of my unborn children that haunted every morning. I felt the same cold draft emanating from the uninhabited nursery next door.

I went off to work, and just as it had yesterday, the routine of the day gradually nudged the pain further and further back into my subconscious. I went to meetings. I worked in the lab. I watched the clock, and it pleasantly surprised me again by making it round to 5:00, just as it had done every other day.

I cooked dinner and ate with James and Marsha. I don't remember what we spoke about. Like I said, it was an ordinary day.

At 7:15 that evening, the phone rang. I leisurely went to get it, with no understanding of how important it would be that I was home to receive this call. I glanced at the caller ID, and was shaken by what I saw. It said "Santa Clara Cty." I knew that calls from the Department of Children and Family Services came with that label.

I took a deep breath and answered the phone.

"Hello," said a woman's voice, "May I please speak with Julie or James Aguas?"

"This is Julie." I blurted out quickly, eager to give the floor back to the voice on the other end.

"Hi Julie. This is Victoria at the Children's Shelter. I'm calling because we have a six month old baby girl here, and we were wondering if you would like to take her home tonight."

A six month old girl! Not the newborn that I longed for, but still very young. I wanted to shout out "Yes! Yes! I'll be there in ten minutes!" and dart out the door, but my common sense kicked in, and I decided to ask at least a few questions.

"Is she free for adoption?" I asked, and closed my eyes trying to mentally transmit the response that I wanted to emerge from Victoria's lips.

"Well this would be an emergency placement at this point. Do you know how concurrent planning works?" She said.

"Yes, I understand." I responded, remembering from Pride class that this meant that there would be simultaneous efforts to reunite her with biological family and secure a fost-adopt plan (which hopefully included me). I needed to get an idea of the risk of the situation. "What do you know about this baby and her situation?" I asked.

"Well, let me see." I heard the sound of shuffling papers. "So it looks like the mother is incarcerated and has already lost other children to the system. All of her other children are in adoptive homes."

It seemed like it would be highly unlikely for the birth mom to reunite with this baby if she was unable to get her act together for the others. That was enough for me to take the plunge. Of course, I needed to run it by James first.

"Would you mind if I spoke to my husband really quickly?" I asked.

"No problem." Victoria responded, "Take your time."

I raced to find James. When I found the bathroom door locked, I pounded on the door.

"Sweetie, Sweetie!" I called breathlessly, "A lady from Children's Shelter is on the phone. There's a six month old baby girl. It sounds like a low-risk situation. There are older siblings, and they have all been adopted. We could go pick her up tonight!"

James, who did not expect to have news like this delivered while sitting on the toilet, said, "Slow down, slow down. We have to think this out." He paused for a second, "Did you ask about the baby? Is she healthy?"

Well that hadn't occurred to me at all. Luckily James was here to do the thinking for the both of us. I went back to Victoria.

"What do you know about the baby? Is she healthy? Has she been exposed to drugs or alcohol?"

"Let me look at the notes." More paper shuffling, "Ok . . . it's a six day old boy. Looks like he's perfectly healthy. He was born negative for drug exposure."

A six day old boy? Wait a second - this kid suddenly got younger and switched genders! I asked Victoria to clarify – was it a six month old girl or a six day old boy? She confirmed that her first statement was the mistake. It was a six day old boy. This could not get any better – a brand new healthy baby with no drug exposure. I relayed this to James, and we both agreed to make an instant beeline for the Children's Shelter. We left the dishes in the sink, and jumped into the car.

I called my mother as soon as we started driving. I could barely get the words out to tell her what was happening. Somehow I must have gotten my point across, since screams of joy were leaping out of the receiver into my ear. Mom immediately dropped everything and ran out to the store to get us diapers, bottles, and whatever other things we would need to get through the first night. At least for tonight, the cosmic powers working against us had taken a hiatus – a baby would be coming home with us!

As we entered Children's Shelter, my eyes darted around, trying to spot the baby. No sign of him. The receptionist summoned Victoria for us, and soon after, a stout woman with dark, loosely tied back hair emerged from a set of cubicles behind the reception area.

"Hi Guys, I'm Victoria." She precariously balanced a stack of papers as she shook our hands, "The worker is on her way with the baby. She'll be here with him in 10 minutes. You can have a seat over there if you'd like. Feel free to turn on the TV."

Aw man, he's not here yet!

More waiting was in store for us. As I turned toward the sitting area, it occurred to me that I had never asked what the baby's name was. I turned back around and asked Victoria before she had a chance to disappear into the maze of cubicles. Victoria adjusted her glasses, and shuffled through the papers in her hands. I braced myself to hear the name. In the Pride class, they had mentioned that it was a common phenomenon for children who ultimately ended up in foster care to be given overly creative names (to put it kindly). We'd heard stories of real kids named Spider, Fantasy, or even Demon. I hoped we would not be spending our first evening with the baby brainstorming a nickname.

"Here it is!" Victoria's head popped out of the stack of papers. I wondered what was in those papers that made it take a full minute to locate a detail as simple as the boy's name. "His name is Jesse."

Jesse. I loved the name Jesse! I had actually suggested that name when James and I were in the midst of our pre-marital baby name negotiations. As I remembered, he had also liked the name, but it had been rejected due to the existence of the female version of the name. We didn't want to give any future bullies ammunition to use against our son. We had eventually settled on Isaac, which we liked as much as the name Jesse, and as far as we knew, did not have any female version.

Now I just needed a face to put with the name. And I needed it soon! Over the past few years, anxious waiting had pretty much become my normal state of being. Surprisingly, despite all the practice, I had not really gotten any better at it. Although the television was on, I did not find that it distracted my intense focus on the happenings out the front window. I kept seeing headlights of cars coming through the parking lot,

The Pursuit of Family

but thus far, there had been no action at the door. The night was cold and stormy. I hoped that there had not been an accident. Nothing was out of the realm of possibility when it came to our bad luck.

At last, a car pulled up directly in front of the entrance. A woman came out of the car, and yes, she was heading to the back seat! This had to be it! She opened the car door, fiddled around for a bit, and soon had an infant seat with a blue blanket draped over it, dangling lightly from her hand.

As she walked in the door, my heart pounded. James and I stood and approached her.

"Are you the foster family?" She asked, smiling.

"Yes," we responded in unison.

"He's a tiny one!" She said as she placed the car seat on the floor and lifted the blanket.

And there he was - all scrunched up in the seat that was at least three times his size. He had a ruddy complexion and deep circles under his eyes. His dimpled chin receded below slightly parted lips which were sucking away at a dreamtime feast. His cheeks had tufts of dark fuzz - the telltale baby sideburns of a preemie. He was wearing the hospital-issue pink and blue beanie on his head and a yellow pajama, both of which swallowed his tiny body.

The moment I caught sight of his old-man face, something deep and primal took hold of my body. My senses heightened and my whole consciousness intensely focused on soaking up every detail of this little being. My eyes locked onto his face, memorizing every contour. I could hear his baby breaths and sighs as though he were right up against my ear. I swear that I could even pick up his sweet scent hanging in the air above him. I was imprinting on him, like a baby bird when it first catches sight of its mother. Deep within me, I felt an instant and fierce love for this magnificent little creation. A white dove may as well have perched on my shoulder dramatically declaring in a James Earl Jones voice, "This is your son."

There was talking going on around me that I was slightly aware of. The social worker handed us a pen, and

A Day Like Any Other

James and I signed a paper which made us Jesse's official foster parents.

"We just need to take him for a quick check-up with the shelter nurse," the social worker said. "Then you can go ahead and take him home."

We went back with him down the hall to the shelter clinic. The nurse came out and peeked into Jesse's seat.

"Oh we have a tiny one, don't we?" She said as she unlatched him and scooped him up. She laid him down on the exam table, and gently removed his clothes. Immediately, his scrawny arms and legs started shaking. A look of panic flashed across his face, and he started screaming. I suppressed my impulse to snatch him from her and protect him from this intrusion. He must have been so cold. He had no fat whatsoever on his body. The skin on his legs sagged like elephant hide.

The nurse quickly looked him over and then weighed him. He was 5 lbs, 5 oz – definitely the smallest baby that I had ever seen up close. She expertly bundled him, despite his flailing limbs. As soon as the last snap was snapped, he was quiet and calm again, like a switch had been flipped. She swaddled him tightly, picked him up off the table, and handed him to me. His warm body relaxed into my arms, and he started to return to sleep. The nurse gave us some instructions, and I tried really hard to listen, resisting the powerful pull to stare some more at the perfect little contents of my arms.

At last, the nurse completed her instructions, and we were free to go. We placed Jesse into the car seat that we had brought, and covered him with the same blue blanket that he came with. I sat next to Jesse in the back seat and admired his face as the shadows danced over him. I knew that there were plenty of things for us to worry about, but they could wait for tomorrow. This was our moment – we were driving home with Baby on Board.

We finally got home with Jesse around midnight. As I pulled him out of his infant seat, James went straight for the camera. My first impulse was to stop him from taking pictures. What if Jesse were taken away from us? Would we want a million pictures of him to remind us of what we once had? I remembered the photos James had taken of my belly from the first pregnancy and how it stung to see those again. Luckily, I stopped myself from saying anything. It was time to live in the moment and put all the fear aside.

And there was no better pull to the moment than the little boy in my arms. I felt like I could just sit and watch his adorably awkward facial expressions all night long. James and I traded turns holding him for a while, and then we decided it was time to put him down to bed. We had a travel-sized bassinette which was more than big enough for our pint-sized guy. He went down with no complaints, and James and I headed straight to bed.

As I lay awake in bed, I listened to his breathing, humming, and cooing. I couldn't wait for him to wake up again. I didn't have to wait long, as he awakened pretty much every hour on the hour for the entire night. As soon as his needs were met though, he would immediately settle into peaceful sleep, the glorious lilt of his breath nourishing my long-starving ears.

Chapter 18
Exposed

The next morning was a Friday, which was a work day. Fortunately, I had thought about this particular situation a lot, and I did have a plan in place for when we got a foster placement. My original plan for when we had a biological baby had been to quit working entirely. But with our situation so tenuous, I feared that if I quit work and ended up losing the baby, I would be left with nothing. A few months back, I had had another epiphany in my usual place of great thinking - the shower. Instead of quitting my job when we got a foster placement, I would cut down to half-time and work from 6:00 – 10:00 in the morning. James would stay home with the baby during that time, and bring him to work at 10:00. At that point, we'd switch off, and James would work from 10:00 am – 7:00 pm. I had already run that by my supervisor, who was a very family-oriented person, and she had agreed to it.

Of course, I wanted some time off with the baby initially before subjecting myself to sleepless nights up with a baby followed by an insanely early morning shift. Sadly, in our country, there is no concept of maternity leave for adoptive parents. Arguably, adoptive parents should get more time off with their new babies since they missed out on the nine months of bonding time that biological parents get. However, maternity leave is not about bonding and is considered to be a purely medical leave. Under the Family Leave Act, adoptive parents do have the right to six weeks of partially paid bonding leave, which biological mothers may take in addition to the regular maternity leave. This leave does not have to be taken in one large chunk and can be spread out over the course of a year. So I decided that I would work from home for one week then take two weeks of vacation. After that, I would return to work on my half-time schedule, using the bonding leave to cover the hours that I was missing from my full-time schedule each day. That way, if we lost Jesse, and somehow, I didn't die in the process, I could seamlessly return to my full-time position.

After settling things at work, I ran Jesse back to the Children's Shelter to visit the doctor. A nurse visit had been sufficient to take him home, but the law required that I take him for a doctor visit as well. Jesse slept in the car as I drove to the shelter. I continually peered out my rearview mirror to try to catch a glimpse of him, but with the rear facing infant seat, it was impossible. I wished that he would cry so that I could be reassured that he was still living and breathing back there. I wondered if I should stop the car and check on him. What if the straps had somehow strangled him? These irrational thoughts probably fly through many mothers' heads, but I would guess that they take up a much more permanent residence in women who have already lost babies. The self-comforting notion that *those unthinkable things* happen to other people, is impossible to subscribe to when the unthinkable actually happens, not just once, but repeatedly. It steals one's ability to feel safe from anything.

At the Children's Shelter, Jesse and I were ushered straight back to the clinic. The nurse who had seen Jesse the night before was there again.

"Oh look, it's little Jesse! How did he do last night?"

"He woke up every hour, but as soon as I fed him, he relaxed really quickly." I said, bursting with pride that my little guy was so easy to calm.

"That's great!" she said as she led us to an exam room, "Let's take off his clothes and get him weighed in."

And the torture ensued. Poor Jesse was still adamantly opposed to undressing. As he screamed and writhed, we weighed him quickly – yep, he was still tiny, just like yesterday. The nurse wrapped him up tightly in a blanket and went to get the doctor.

The doctor came in shortly and reinitiated Jesse's screaming as she opened up the blanket. She did the basic exam – pretty much the same as the nurse had done the night before, listening to his heart, looking in his ears, and moving around his limbs.

"Jesse has a lot of extra muscle tone, especially in his legs," the doctor commented.

"Yeah, he seems like such a strong baby," I said, beaming, "He's already able to hold his head up pretty well." A vision flashed in my mind of Jesse on the podium receiving his first Olympic gold.

The brass ensemble in my brain had just reached "the dawn's early light" when the doctor interrupted, "Actually, we shouldn't be seeing that kind of muscle tone in an infant. Babies are supposed to be kind of soft and floppy. He is a little on the stiff side."

What are you getting at? Is there something wrong with Jesse?

"This is what we expect to see with drug exposure," she nonchalantly stated.

"But he tested negative for drugs." I responded, certain that she was mistaken.

"Yes, but drugs will only show up in the baby's urine if the mom had used within three days of his birth. She was in jail, so she couldn't have. However, it is probable that she used drugs during the pregnancy. And they actually do the most damage in the early months when the brain and other organs are forming. This would also explain his very short sleep intervals."

My stomach turned at the thought of this precious baby being poisoned before he was even born.

"How will this affect his development?" I asked, steadying myself against the exam table.

"The muscle tone will probably normalize over time" the doctor responded, "But the long-term effects of drug exposure vary from child to child. He may have behavior problems, learning problems, physical problems, or he may be totally normal. It's impossible to predict. He is a healthy baby at this point, and you are giving him the best start possible."

As I dressed Jesse, I looked into his sharply alert eyes. The energy that projected from them was unmistakable. I had no doubt in my mind that Jesse was bright, socially connected, and strong. That would be all that he would need to overcome whatever limitations the drug exposure may place on him. He would heal from this just as James and I would heal from all the poison that life had injected into our veins. As long as we were together, we could get through anything.

As long as we were together – the terror induced by that statement so crowded my consciousness that any concerns about drug exposure seemed about as weighty as a hangnail. James and I were already so madly in love with this baby that we knew we could face any issue that he could possibly have. But losing him was another story – that would surely kill us.

My days with Jesse were a constant juxtaposition of pure joy and agonizing worry. Caring for Jesse was more intensely satisfying than I had ever imagined. As I went about doing ordinary household chores, I would suddenly detect a huge grin plastered across my face just at the thought of the magnificent boy snoozing in the next room. When I held him, every micro-expression that appeared on his face provided unparalleled entertainment. There was nothing in life that could compare to the feeling of each baby breath as he warmly nuzzled in sleep against me, completely form-fitting to my body.

I began to notice that my general aversion to babies had vanished. I found myself peeking into the baby carriages of strangers and smiling – something I had not done in years. I no longer hated the women pushing the baby carriages either and could have painless interactions with them, provided that they weren't pregnant. The sight of a pregnant belly was still like a knife to the chest, but at least babies themselves no longer elicited a painful response – one segment of the population that I could happily re-integrate into my life.

But during the quiet moments when I was not under the influence of Jesse's blissful intoxication, the panic would set in. It was especially punctuated by the severe sleep deprivation that was accumulating with each passing, sleepless night. From time to time, I would just collapse into the vision of the worst-case scenario. Jesse is taken away. My work life is upside down. We are unable to produce a biological child and too emotionally scarred to face another failed adoption. Our marriage falls apart. Everything is lost.

Jesse's social worker had explained to me over the phone all of the very real scenarios in which we could lose Jesse. One would be if the biological father were found. He or one of his relatives might want Jesse, and they would have priority over us. So far, they hadn't been able to locate the alleged father, and even if they did, there was no guarantee that his DNA would confirm him as the father. The other, even more possible scenario was if one of the adoptive parents of Jesse's half-siblings wanted Jesse. They would have priority over us as well. So far, none of them had been contacted, so that remained hanging over our heads. Even if none of those scenarios came to pass, we still were not guaranteed to be matched with Jesse as his fost-adopt family. The fact that we had him now gave us an edge over other families, but if there was a family that the team felt matched Jesse better than us, they could choose them over us. So once again, we found ourselves with our emotional survival precariously dangling from a fragile tree branch in the gusty air above us, well beyond our reach.

Jesse's sleep situation had not been good from the start. He could only sleep for very short intervals at a time – usually one to two hours at night and 20 minutes during the day. He had become adamantly opposed to sleeping in a crib or bassinet, and the only way we could get him to sleep was in his bouncy chair that vibrated. We had replaced the battery on that puppy at least a dozen times already!

When Jesse was about three weeks old, the sleep situation dramatically worsened. He started waking up at night with glass-shattering shrieks that didn't even sound human. James and I would try to hold and comfort him, but his body would get very stiff and start arching backwards. He would sweat and writhe as though he were in serious pain. I'm sure the floors in our house had never seen more foot traffic in their 60 years of existence as during that time of nightly pacing through the house with our distressed infant. We fed him, bounced him, swaddled him tightly, and positioned him every which way, continuously praying that something would do the trick to calm him. We tried walking him through the house in his stroller and driving him around in the car. This actually made him more upset. When he would finally fall asleep, we would carefully transfer him back into his bouncy chair. Nine out of ten times, that would wake him and start the whole process over again. And the one lucky time in ten tries, our painstaking efforts would only give us at most a two hour reprieve before we were back on duty.

It was right about this time that my leave ran out, and I returned to work on my brilliantly planned early morning schedule. By this point, the sleep deprivation had become so severe that I was frequently having trouble getting words out to form a coherent sentence. My thinking was completely jumbled, and my worries were multiplied by a factor of about a thousand. Jesse's pediatrician had given us no insights except to say that the nervous system of a drug-exposed child is very sensitive. During the long nights, from time to time I would feel a surge of irrational anger toward Jesse. I would look at him as he screamed and think, "Why are you doing this to me? Just shut up and sleep!" Directing these horrible thoughts toward an innocent, suffering baby made me feel like a completely inadequate mother.

When the schedule of county-sponsored classes for foster parents came out, James and I were thrilled to find out that they were offering a course on Parenting the Drug-Exposed Child. We attended the class, hopeful that it would provide the magic formula for calming Jesse. The presenter spoke at length about the numerous, terrifying issues that we may or may not face in the future, but didn't spend any time on infant sleep issues. When it came time for questions, my hand shot up, and I described Jesse's sleep issues. The presenter suggested that we swaddle him tightly, prevent him from arching his back, and bounce him - all things that we were already doing. Luckily, among the handouts from the class was a description of infant massage, which I decided might do some good for Jesse. At least we were leaving with something new to try.

As we were preparing to leave, a woman approached us. I immediately recognized her as someone we had previously met in our CPR class. Her name was Kristina, and she and her husband had been doing emergency foster care for the past few years since their three biological daughters were grown. They had fostered 30 children thus far! In fact, she was holding number 30 in her arms. He was the same age as Jesse and also having issues due to drug exposure. She described a special cradle called the Nature's Cradle which was helping her little boy to sleep better. She offered to try to locate one for us, so we exchanged contact information.

The next day, we received an email from Kristina, giving us the phone number of a foster mother named Shelly who had a Nature's Cradle and was finished using it. I quickly contacted Shelly and set up a time that evening for us to pick it up.

Shelly answered the door with a gorgeous three-month old baby boy in her arms who I presumed was the graduate of the cradle. The baby greeted us with a smile as we entered the home.

"So here is the cradle," Shelly motioned toward the center of the family room, "I hope you have room in your car."

The Nature's Cradle was quite a sight to behold. Standing about waist high, it somewhat resembled the bassinets that hospitals use for infants. A sturdy, wheeled base supported a white, rectangular cradle which was about six inches deep. At the foot of the cradle was a control panel with several knobs and buttons. A frilly white bed-skirt beneath the cradle piece attempted to disguise the fact that this contraption was a heavy duty piece of machinery – sort of like putting a dress on a pro wrestler. I didn't care what it looked like though as long as it did its job to lull Jesse into dreamland.

The cradle was mounted on hydraulics which allowed it to not simply rock, but move in every direction. In this way, it simulated the motions of the mother which the baby had grown accustomed to while inside the womb. The motion varied in intensity, and speakers underneath the mattress played the sound of a heartbeat which sped up and slowed down in time with the motion of the cradle. That thing really moved – I was getting sea-sick just watching it. You could set the cradle to simulate daytime movements or nighttime movements. Also, it had a setting for the age of the baby. As the baby got older, the cradle would be still more of the time so that the baby would be gradually weaned off of the motion. Impressive.

As we talked with Shelly, we found out that the baby boy she was holding was their second fost-adopt child. His older sister, who was 18 months old, was down the hall getting bathed by Daddy. The children were half-siblings, and they were both heavily drug-exposed. I described what we were going through with Jesse.

"That is exactly what it was like for us," said Shelly. "I found out when we were going through it that the meth is stored in their fat cells, and it takes about three weeks after they're born for it to be expelled from the body. At that point is when the withdrawals begin."

That explained why Jesse was suddenly getting worse! I wondered why no doctor had ever mentioned this to me.

"How long did the withdrawals last for your kids?" I asked, unsure if I really wanted to hear the answer or not.

"For our kids, they lasted about a month."

Wow. I shuddered to think of Jesse's suffering and our sleep deprivation continuing for an entire month.

"But I can tell you this," Shelly continued, "There are few experiences that so tightly bond parents and children like going through withdrawals together."

Reflecting upon her statement, I realized that she was right. Our bond with Jesse had exponentially intensified since the withdrawals had started. Our protective instincts for him were on high alert, and he was learning that we could be trusted to stick with him through the worst of times. A month is a long period of time. And experiencing all 30 days as well as nights in wakefulness effectively doubles the length of the wait. However, despite the failings of many forces in my life that I once counted on, I knew that time would fulfill its promise to continue passing. We would get though this, and we would come out of it stronger.

Just then a flash of long wet hair darted across the family room. Shelly's daughter had emerged from her bath. She was a petite girl with a ton of hair and a smile that was bigger than she was. Shelly's husband, David came out as well and greeted us. The four of them made a beautiful family. They had bonds that transcended biology. They had battled in the darkest of trenches together and had emerged victorious.

Shelly and her husband gave us several other tips. They showed us the padded wedge they used to make their son feel cozy in the Nature's Cradle. They showed us the special bottles they used which were tall and narrow, with a smaller nipple and a straw inside which released the air in the space above the milk. This design made it easier for babies to feed and reduced gas. We hoped that these bottles would make a big difference for Jesse since he spit up pretty much constantly. We learned so much more from a half-hour with real parents than we did in the three-hour class!

The Nature's Cradle just barely fit into the back of our SUV. It was a lucky thing because it didn't look like it could be disassembled for transport. We brought it home and placed it next to Jesse's crib. Since Jesse still preferred to sleep in a sitting position, we decided that he should take his maiden test-drive of the cradle in his car seat. The car seat in which he was already sleeping fit perfectly and securely in the cradle box. So we placed him in and turned it on. He remained peacefully sleeping and we tiptoed out, fingers crossed.

During the night, Jesse still woke us up with screams that rattled the light fixtures. He still stiffened and arched and struggled as he exorcised the demons the drugs had left in his weary body. But we did notice that with the new cradle, his sleep intervals were now approaching two hours, and when we put him back to bed, he more often relaxed into the cradle rather than waking up. The mere fact that we now knew what his problem was and approximately how long it would last made the nights much more bearable.

I had also started to do infant massage with Jesse each evening. At first his skin was very sensitive, and I couldn't do much more than his legs. Gradually, he began to enjoy the massages more and more. It was a wonderful time that we spent together. He would relax and babble at me and shoot me a smile from time to time. Even though he still constantly spit up, he must have been getting some food down because his scrawny body was quickly chubbing up. His saggy, baggy leg skin now wrapped firmly around the beginnings of healthy rolls of fat. His old man face was now rounded out by irresistibly plump baby cheeks. Seeing him growing and thriving eased the pain of the long nights.

Chapter 19
Farewell to Convention

By early February all of the test results had come back from the fourth miscarriage, and it was time to see Dr. Locke for a consult. This time, James and I did not have to rely on real estate magazines to occupy our minds while waiting. We had a lovely baby boy with us. As we were ushered to the consultation room, the nurses all went nuts over the tiny guy in my arms.

When Dr. Locke arrived, she was surprised to see us with a baby. We explained to her how Jesse had come into our lives. She seemed relieved, as though the impact of the news that she was about to deliver would be softened by his presence.

Dr. Locke sat down in the chair across from us and took a deep breath. "So the karyotype results came back Normal, Female. We consider this result to be inconclusive since we can't be sure that it wasn't your tissue that was tested. But the likelihood is that the cause of this miscarriage was the same cause as the previous ones, which is unexplained. Many of these unexplained cases are actually immunological problems that are not well understood. One thing that sometimes works for patients like this is to use donor sperm or a donor egg. If your immune system has identified a particular set of DNA to attack, then using different DNA can sometimes prevent the attack. Other than that, there is no more treatment that I can offer you."

I was not ready to consider using donor egg or sperm.

"But this last pregnancy went further than any other has gone." I pleadingly stated, "Doesn't that mean that the

Lovenox did something? Couldn't we just increase the dosage?"

"Lovenox also acts as an immunosuppressant. So that may explain why it helped somewhat in this case. Increasing the dosage, however, would be dangerous to you and the baby. We're at the absolute maximum for your weight."

I thought back over my many research sessions on the Internet. I remembered reading about immunological treatments for miscarriage. There was a lot of controversy surrounding them, but they did exist. I brought this up to Dr. Locke.

"Yes, there are some immunological treatments, but they are quite expensive and they have not been proven effective." She paused momentarily, as if unsure whether or not to continue. "There is a doctor in Los Gatos. I don't know if you've heard of him. His name is Adam Brewer."

"I think I've heard the name, but I don't know anything about him." I replied.

"Well, some of our patients continue on with him after all conventional options are exhausted."

"Have they been successful?" I asked.

"Some are and some aren't." Dr. Locke replied, "But just because some succeed on his treatments doesn't mean that they wouldn't have been successful anyway without the treatments. There are really no medical studies to prove that his treatments work any better than doing absolutely nothing."

At this point, my belief in conventional medicine for treating miscarriage was right on a par with my belief in the Easter Bunny. Unconventional was the only way to go. At least we had not reached a complete dead end. I was not ready to give up yet. So I called Dr. Brewer's office that day and set the wheels in motion for us to meet with him. I transferred my never-ending novel of medical records over to him and completed a laundry list of blood tests that he required. I hoped that some piece of information we were sending him would hold the key to identifying the cause of our reproductive woes.

As we waited for our consult, I continued to get to know Jesse. One thing became exceedingly clear to me early on – Jesse loved to be held. I loved to hold Jesse, so it made for a good match. I figured that the more I held him, the more our bond would solidify. And I strongly wanted to somehow make up for the nine months when another woman was holding him. However, there were one or two (or more like a hundred) things that I needed to do around the house which were difficult to do without the use of my arms. Either I could adapt and become more dexterous with my feet, or I could buy some sort of baby carrier. Opting for the latter, I purchased a baby sling that draped over one shoulder and held Jesse snuggly across my abdomen.

Jesse thoroughly approved of the purchase. Nothing made him happier than lounging in his cozy Mommy-supported hammock. Every time I put him in, he would instantly calm down and drift off to sleep. In fact, I found that if I kept him in there, I could actually get him to sleep one to two consecutive hours rather than the 15-20 minute snoozes he normally took. By placing him in the sling at regular intervals, I was able to simulate a nap schedule. Jesse savored the snuggling, and I could work around the house as he slept. Of course, he would soon be getting too large to carry in this manner, so this solution was temporary. I hoped that if his body got trained to sleeping on a schedule, it would be easier to get him to desire the same napping schedule outside of the sling.

We brought Jesse in his sling to our first visit at the Brewer Clinic. We got some funny looks from the staff and the patients in the waiting room. I don't think people expected to see a woman with a tiny infant seeking the care of a top fertility expert.

I had researched Dr. Brewer after leaving Dr. Locke's office, and he was truly a living legend. He was the lone pioneer of reproductive immunology which was a rapidly growing, though widely criticized field. Through a lifetime of research, Dr. Brewer was able to unravel the insanely complex immune system to identify many of the main culprits behind reproductive failure. He had also developed treatments to counteract them, which had reportedly helped countless couples to overcome their infertility.

I had never before met someone who had pioneered a field of medicine. I didn't know what to expect when the nurse dropped us off at the door of Dr. Brewer's small office. Would he be a bowtie-clad, inaccessible scholar? Or maybe some kind of a wild-haired mad scientist like Doc Brown in <u>Back To the Future</u>?

A friendly voice ushered us in. Contrary to any of my guesses, Dr. Brewer looked more like a sweet old grandpa. He was casually dressed and wore the deep lines of a lifetime of caring smiles. He sat us down and first sincerely expressed his sympathy for all that we had been through. He told us that these problems are not our fault, and that we are not alone in our struggles. He locked his gaze firmly on my watery eyes said with great conviction, "I know that I can help you."

This was the first time that a doctor had been more than just clinical with us – the first time a doctor had filled us with a sense of confidence and allowed us to rest our faith on his sturdy shoulders. I really appreciated this approach. Whether or not he really could help us, at least I felt propped up by his strength and whole-hearted support.

Next he stepped us through our test results, explaining each test and the meaning of the results. First off, a genetic marker called the DQ alpha had been tested. My DQ alpha was 501, which he said was the mark of a particularly powerful immune system. Most of the time, that is a good thing because people with the 501 marker are typically super healthy, like I was. I never had been one to get sick my entire life. I also had a history of getting high fevers after tetanus shots and flu vaccines which indicated that my immune system was particularly overzealous.

Dr. Brewer informed us that three of my test results were out of line with normal. At long last, I had flunked!! I had too few blocking antibodies, which serve as a shield to prevent the immune system from attacking the fetus. The activation of my natural killer (NK) cells was too high, which could potentially cause an attack on the growing placenta. Lastly, Dr. Brewer believed that my MTHFR mutation indicated a clotting disorder, even though the other doctors had considered it a normal result.

I mentioned to him that my other doctors had said that over 40% of the population had that mutation and that it was not significant.

Dr. Brewer's manner suddenly changed. He glared at me and began to raise his voice. "I have seen a perfectly healthy woman with the same mutation give birth at 39 weeks gestation and promptly die of a stroke."

It was clear to me at that point that this particular living legend did not like to be questioned, so I shut up and listened. His voice reverted back to the caring, sympathetic tone as he explained the treatments that we would do to counteract these problems. I would take a medicine called Enbrel for a month or so to bring down the activation of the NK cells. James and I would do a treatment called LIT to bring up the blocking antibodies. This treatment involved injecting a component of James' blood under the skin on my arms. He said to think of it as an immunization. Once all of my levels came back to normal, I would be cleared for a cycle. To counteract the clotting disorder, I would take Lovenox injections and baby aspirin throughout the entire pregnancy. We would continue to test the NK cell activation at set intervals during the pregnancy, and as soon as it ever became high again, I would do a treatment called IVIG to bring it back down. I liked this active approach of monitoring and treating the pregnancy. In the past, our only indication of how things were going was to check on the ultrasound if the baby was dead yet. Now we would be able to catch and counteract the culprit before the damage was done.

Dr. Brewer started to draw a timeline of my cycle on a sheet of paper. "You will begin taking Clomid on day three of your cycle. Then start the Lovenox and baby aspirin on day six." He marked the timeline as he spoke. "Your gynecologist can track the growth of your follicles, and when you have a mature follicle, you will start having intercourse." I inwardly chuckled as he marked his diagram with little hearts. "Then two days later, take the hcg injection."

After putting the finishing touches on the timeline, Dr. Brewer got a glimmer in his eyes. "Do you want to see the cover of my book? I am getting it published soon, and the cover just came in."

Dr. Brewer's excitement over his book was quite endearing. As we admired the cover, the breadth of his grin could have rivaled the Cheshire Cat.

"I can't wait to read it when it comes out." I said.

"I'm going to go on Oprah soon too." Dr. Brewer beamed with delight.

"Wow!" I replied. "That is really exciting. I will definitely tune in for that!"

We were certainly in the big leagues now. Our doctor was going to appear on Oprah! If he couldn't help us, I didn't know who could.

As we left Dr. Brewer's office, he told us to go to the nurse for further instructions. The nurse first told us how we could go about getting Enbrel, giving us a list of possible pharmacies. Our insurance would probably not cover it, just as it probably would not cover today's consult with Dr. Brewer. She next explained with a completely nonchalant tone that since the FDA had recently banned the LIT treatment, we would have to travel to Mexico in order to receive it.

Wait a second, what? Did I hear that right? We have to cross the border and go to some God-knows-how-legitimate clinic in order to receive a medical treatment that was banned in the United States? How crazy do you think we are?

The nurse handed us the contact information for a clinic in Nogales, Mexico. I had to stop her there. "Umm, why did the FDA ban LIT?"

"They felt that the studies didn't support its effectiveness. Even though LIT is completely safe, the FDA has become very particular about treatments which involve the sharing of blood products. You can read Dr. Brewer's rebuttal online. The studies which were done were very poorly constructed. This treatment is safe and effective. We did it for years in this office. And Dr. Brewer personally trained the doctor in Nogales who performs it, so he knows what he is doing."

I still felt uneasy. I knew that reproductive immunology was a bit off of the beaten path of conventional medicine, but this was a leap miles away from my field of vision of the path. The nurse continued to give instructions, but my mind was still stuck on this crossing the border business. When she finished, we paid for the consult, and turned in a state of shock to exit the clinic.

A woman approached us who had been sitting in the lobby as we were speaking to the nurse.

"I felt the same way when I first heard about having to go to Nogales, but I did it back in January, and it's really no big deal."

"Really?" I said. "It totally freaks me out."

"Don't worry. It's a piece of cake. Dr. Quiroz is really great. And, hey it worked for me so far. I'm on my way to my first ultrasound, and so far, I'm doing great."

"Oh, congratulations!" I said.

"Here, I'll give you my email address, and I can tell you all of the specifics and answer any questions you have."

I was filled with a rush of gratitude not only for getting some reassurance from a real live survivor of this bizarre treatment, but also to meet someone in the flesh who was in the midst of the same struggle as me. This was the first time I had made contact with a single soul on the planet who was currently trudging through life in a pair of really crappy shoes similar to my own. I at once felt sure that I could handle this course of treatment. After all, the only other choice I had was to give up, and that was not a part of my vocabulary.

I looked down at little Jesse, who was sleeping peacefully in my sling. Maybe all of our struggles so far were somehow set in motion so that we could fulfill our destiny of being united with Jesse. Now that we were together, maybe everything would just fall into place for us to have a biological child.

My email correspondence with the lady from the clinic began right away. Her name was Maya, and her first email to me told the story of her two miscarriages and one ectopic pregnancy that led her to Dr. Brewer. It told of the details of the Nogales trip. She and her husband were instructed to arrive at a McDonald's on the Arizona side of Nogales early in the morning. There they met with all of the other couples who were going for LIT the same day. An employee of the clinic fetched them all at the McDonald's and led them on foot across the border to the clinic. They were instructed to carry $600 cash to pay for the treatment. The only things this story was missing were code names and secret handshakes! At the clinic, the doctor took blood from Maya's husband, and then after processing the blood, did the injections into Maya's arm. Maya said that it stung, but wasn't too bad. Then they came back over the border, and it was over. The results so far were very good – Maya's ultrasound had gone great. They saw the heartbeat and everything looked perfect. I knew that at only six weeks, she was nowhere near out of the woods in terms of miscarriage, but so far so good.

    I felt confident enough at this point to sign up with the clinic for an LIT treatment in early April. I booked our tickets and arranged for lodging in Tucson, Arizona. We would do the fastest trip possible, arriving in Tucson the afternoon prior to the LIT and leaving the following afternoon right after the treatment was over. Since Jesse was only a foster child at this point, we knew that crossing the border with him was probably not the best idea. We had visions of being accused of baby-smuggling on the way back to the States since Jesse was of Mexican ethnicity, and we had no official documents for him. So we arranged for him to stay with my mother while we were gone. James and I hated to think about separating from him at all, but we could all survive for one night. In fact, the one obvious perk was that James and I might actually get our first full night of uninterrupted sleep.

Chapter 20
Happy Birthday

About a week after our visit with Dr. Brewer, I was forced to say goodbye to another precious thing that I longed to hold on to – my 20s. Yes, I had hit the big 3-0, and there was no turning back. How different my life was than I had expected it would be at 30. According to my life plan, which had been laid out before I had even seen my 20s, I would have been married at 22. I would have had my first baby at 23 and my second at 25. So if things had gone as I had planned, I would have had two children in elementary school at this point.

As my plan had specified, I did have two children at this point - an infant and a highschooler. I was sure they were every bit as wonderful as my imagined 5 and 7 year olds. But my life was quite different from my neat little plan. Each morning I wondered if my son would still be mine by the evening. Each time the phone rang, I would approach the receiver like the bomb squad approaches a ticking suitcase. Would this be the call that haunted my nightmares?

And according to my plan, I would be done having children at this point. I would be settled into an easy routine of raising them and delighting in them. But I was not done. My heart still ached for the experience of pregnancy and childbirth, so until that happened, my life would feel unsettled. I always felt that I wouldn't mind hitting particular ages as long as I was where I expected to be at that point in my life. I wanted nothing more than to feel settled and comfortable, and I was about as far from that as I could be.

For me, each passing year also represented a further decline in fertility. With my reproductive system as pathetic as it was in my 20s, how bad would it be now that I was in my 30s?

So I made my family promise not to acknowledge my birthday in any way shape or form. It was just too depressing for me. And as per my request, the day of my birthday came and went like any other day.

The next day, James approached me in the family room.

"I did what you wanted and didn't mention your birthday yesterday. But I need to mark the occasion in some way. Happy Birthday Sweetheart."

James handed me a DVD. I looked at the words scribbled with Sharpee pen across the top face - "Happy B-day Julie! From: Hubby".

"What is this?" I said smiling, completely intrigued as to what the mysterious DVD held beneath its shiny surface.

"Well, put it in and play it." James instructed.

I placed it in the DVD player and turned on the TV. I started to hear the gentle plucking of a guitar. Words appeared on the screen explaining that the DVD was going to attempt to capture who I am through the eyes of the people who love me. I sat down and a pool of tears immediately started collecting in my transfixed eyes. How did James have time to put this all together?

The first to appear was Marsha. She spoke, completely unscripted, about how she feels about me and how I've helped her in her life. How many 14 year olds would be able to freely pour out their hearts in front of a camera like that? I could not imagine a more loving child. The words that Marsha spoke were exactly what I needed to hear at this moment. I had been feeling so badly about how the constant drama in my life had hijacked my attention away from her. As a young teenager, this was when she needed me operating at full capacity more than ever! But as she spoke, I felt the warmth of Marsha's genuine appreciation for me, faults and all. She even started to tear up at the end. At this point, my tears were careening down my face in every which way. The tissue manufacturers were certainly going to profit from each viewing of this DVD!

Next a montage of pictures of Marsha started popping onto the screen. It began with her as a very small child, and as birthday parties, family outings, and school events flashed onto the screen, Marsha grew before my eyes. Just the way it happened in real life – it all went by so quickly.

Next the handsome director of the film appeared and talked about his love for me. I flashed back to the moment that he proposed to me those years ago on the pier. He had spoken in the same sweet and genuine way at that time – not a flowery, fake speech written to impress a panel of literature critics, but a simple birds-eye view into his heart. There was nothing that anyone could have done to make me feel more loved and special than I did at that moment.

As I continued to sniffle, the movie continued with images of our dates, silly pranks, Halloween parties at work, and other special memories together. As tragic as our marriage had been so far, I had to marvel at all of the fun that we had in the midst of the struggle.

The mood of the film grew somber as the words on the screen told of some dark times, and the images showed a couple vacationing in Carmel with the light gone from their eyes. But as the images continued, the smiles gradually and miraculously re-emerged.

Suddenly the music turned upbeat as the Fleetwood Mac song, "Don't Stop Thinking About Tomorrow" started to play. The words then told of how perseverance can lead to miracles. And at that moment the weary face of a six-day-old baby appeared on the screen. The emotion of this moment was overwhelming. I looked at the beautiful baby on the screen and realized how much he had changed just in the short time we'd had him. A video clip played of him turning to look at us. The moment he caught sight of us, his mouth exploded into a smile, and he squeaked with joy. He was our miracle, our resurrection from the ashes of the past.

The final montage was of our entire family – my parents, my grandparents, my brother, James' family, my nieces and nephews. All of the people whose love I had felt propping me up through the downfall of these past few years.

For that moment, I felt like the most blessed person in the world. I hugged my magnificent husband and thanked him for this amazing gift. Despite all of the reasons it shouldn't be, he had given me a happy birthday.

Chapter 21
A Run for the Border

Ever since we had gotten Jesse, the weather had been quite stormy – a very long stretch without the sun for California. The first time I noticed the sun peeking out of the clouds after several months of absence, I looked down at the stroller I was pushing and joked,

"Look Jesse, that's what we call the sun. I know you've never seen it before, but isn't it nice?"

The brightening of the weather was a welcome change, but it also signaled the immanence of our trip to Nogales. James and I were dreading the separation from Jesse. Our fertility problems had caused such a long wait to get a baby, and now they were causing separation from the baby that we finally had.

On the day of our departure, we loaded our phones with pictures of our beautiful boy and lingered with him as long as we could at the airport before we parted to meet our plane. I felt a dull ache as I walked away from him. This trip could not be over soon enough.

The weather in Tucson was also pleasant – dry, but pleasant. As we headed for the hotel, we admired the barren, yet strangely breathtaking view. All varieties of cactus dotted the landscape, and in the distance, dramatic, sharp-angled rock mountains lined the horizon.

My one silver lining to the trip, the uninterrupted night of sleep, never came to pass. The night was spent waking up at the regular intervals to which I had become accustomed, even in the absence of a crying baby. I much preferred waking to a real live baby than to a programmed memory of one.

We arose at 5:00 to set off for Nogales. The drive was as simple as it gets. There was only one road, so there was no way to get lost. I'm sure the simplicity of the route was an intentional way to prevent illegal entrants into the country – only one road upon which to set up a checkpoint. I remarked how something that simplifies life for those traveling one direction can seriously complicate life for those traveling the other way.

We easily found the McDonalds that had been described to us. As we entered, we looked around. How were we going to recognize the other couples that we were supposed to meet? We scanned the room. There were other couples there, but they all had the air of confidence that they were in the right place. We were looking for people who appeared as confused and ill at ease as we were. Finally a couple entered the door with a searching expression of wide-eyed apprehension. We approached them, and sure enough, they shared in our quest for the outlawed medical procedure.

We chatted with them, and exchanged fertility woes. It turned out that they had been trying to get pregnant for over five years. They had done multiple rounds of very costly in vitro fertilization with no success. They were originally from Indonesia and currently lived in Michigan. They had done a long distance consult with Dr. Brewer. He found that they landed in every single category of immunological reproduction problems – low blocking antibodies, thrombophilia, antinuclear antibodies, antisperm antibodies and lymphocytes. I wasn't sure what all of these were, but I remembered that Dr. Brewer had mentioned that our problems spanned three categories of immunological problems. So I supposed we weren't the worst possible case.

Other couples gradually started pouring in. We all introduced each other and started to share our stories. There was Abby and her partner who had lost a baby at 16 weeks and then had not been able to get pregnant since. Matt and Lorraine had been trying unsuccessfully to get pregnant for five years, even transferring eight embryos in one IVF cycle, and had never even registered a faint positive pregnancy test.

There was Roma and her husband who had been through three early miscarriages. Chloe and her husband had suffered two early miscarriages. Kate and her husband had tried for ages to get pregnant, had raised a family of foster children to adulthood, and were still trying. Laura and her husband had been trying for 15 years to get pregnant without any luck. Laura was 47 years old. Debby and Fred had a biological son together with no problem, but then had been trying for a second baby for six years. Jenn, like me, had also had four early miscarriages. It appeared that we were the record holders for that dubious distinction.

After we had been chatting for a few minutes, an employee from the clinic arrived and led us across the border. I scanned the surroundings as I walked. The streets of Nogales bustled with activity. Vendors sold snacks and colorful trinkets. Sweaty children ran around in tank tops and flip flops. Various people sat under the cover of awnings, vigorously fanning their otherwise motionless bodies. I felt rather vulnerable being herded through the streets in a conspicuous group of Americans, each of whom carried $600 in cash.

Dr. Quiroz's office was located in a two story, bright blue building. We followed our guide up the stairs.

One of the ladies commented, "In the picture I saw of this clinic on the Internet, it was painted pink."

"Maybe it's color coded," I joked, "If the building is blue when you come, you'll have a boy, and pink, you'll have a girl."

Laura chuckled, "What are you hoping to have?"

"I couldn't care less as long as it's human." I responded.

Lorraine chimed in, "I'm flexible on the human part as long as I can give birth to it."

We all nodded, understanding all too well that sentiment.

Upon arriving in the office, we checked in and paid up. We were briefed on the process. The husbands would first have their blood drawn. Then there would be a two to three hour wait while the blood was processed. During that time, we were free to grab lunch and then return to have the processed blood injected back under the skin of the ladies' forearms.

While the husbands took turns getting their blood drawn, we all sat and talked. People shared horror stories of obtuse doctors, painful procedures, and decimated dreams. Every person in the room had been forever changed by their battle with this all-consuming curse. In daily life, they, like me were all finding it impossible to move their thoughts toward anything besides the horror of their experience and the plan to reach their goal.

The pain of Abby's struggle was etched into her eyes. Her anger wound tightly around her vocal chords as she spoke, "One of the toughest things for me is that I've lost so many friends. They all keep having kids, one by one. They don't understand what I'm going through, and they are constantly so insensitive. I just decided not to subject myself to associating with them anymore."

The group collectively affirmed Abby's mindset. I felt a huge release of pent-up guilt when I realized that I was not the only person in the world suffering from the soul-damning curse of baby envy. I was not the only one who went to great efforts to weasel my way out of baby showers. I was not the only one who isolated myself from the world of blissful mothers, shamefully enumerating the reasons that I would make a better mother than they. In fact, the more we spoke, I discovered that some of these women were perhaps even more bitter and jaded than I was.

Although a deep chasm stood between me and the Sisterhood of women who have undergone the miracle of pregnancy and childbirth, I was not left without a Sisterhood of my own. We were a sorority that no one would voluntarily join, but we were bonded nonetheless in our complete understanding of each other's warped ways. Outsiders could never begin to fathom the fire within us that relentlessly burned, scorching us inside and fueling our every motivation.

A couple of the women lamented that Dr. Brewer was the end of their road. If this treatment didn't work, they would cut their losses and move on to adoption. I found that a good moment to share with the group our adoption journey, from the nightmare of Kelsey to the pure joy of Jesse. Many of the women had clearly been pondering adoption for a while. They jumped on the opportunity to get our opinions on the pros and cons of public adoption. I was glad to have a success story to share for a change to give others hope.

Lorraine pleadingly asked, "Does it still hurt every time you see a baby?"

I honestly responded. "When Jesse is with me, it is a million times easier to see other babies. I wish I could say the same for pregnant women, but that is still just as painful."

Lorraine started to cry, "I wish that I could take that step, but I don't feel like I could wholeheartedly move on to adoption until I had fully given up on carrying my own baby."

The last man emerged, applying pressure to his arm. We were now free to go to lunch. Fred and Debby, who had already been to Nogales for an LIT treatment several weeks before, said that they had discovered a nice place to eat. So they led us down the street, across train tracks to a unique restaurant that was built right into a cliff-side. Inside, a Mariachi band played a lively staccato tune. The tablecloths and wall decorations were vibrant weavings of green and red. This contrasted the gray, stone face of the mountain that served as one of the four walls.

The lunch conversation was much lighter. Tragedy and bouncy Mariachi music just don't make sense together. We spoke of our careers, our pets, and our homes – the normal side of our lives. It was pleasant, and the food was quite good.

We returned to the clinic satisfied with our meal and ready to get the treatment over with. The assistant called our names one by one. When it was my turn, James and I entered Dr. Quiroz's office together. It was a small office, cluttered with pictures of what I presumed was the doctor's family. I chuckled as I noticed that the whole display seemed a bit dwarfed by an 8x10 portrait of Dr. Brewer. James, being fluent in Spanish, greeted Dr. Quiroz, and the two exchanged small-talk. Gesturing toward the photos, Dr. Quiroz mentioned to James that he owed his family to Dr. Brewer, who had treated his wife as well. I supposed that I would want to display a portrait of the good doctor in every room of my house if he could work the same magic on me.

After checking my identity against the writing on the syringe, Dr. Quiroz did not waste any time, grabbing my arm and holding it tightly. He rapidly plunged the needle into my forearm and injected the clear fluid. The moment he would pull the needle out, he would jab it back into another spot on my stunned, defenseless arm. My teeth latched tightly to my lower lip in an attempt to distract from the stab and burn ritual going on below. He repeated the process on the other arm. However shocking, the entire thing was all over within 30 seconds. It was not my idea of a fun Saturday activity, but it was also not the most painful thing I'd ever experienced.

And with that, we were free to go. Not a moment too soon, since the timing was getting tight for us to catch our flight home. We exchanged contact information with our newfound kindred spirits, said goodbye, and raced out of the bright blue building back to the border.

Getting across the border in the reverse direction was much more arduous. James, my throbbing arms, and I stood in a line that wound down the street with no overhang to protect us from the intense midday sun. I was wearing a long sleeved shirt as per the doctor's orders against sun exposure to the welts on my arms. Sweat pushed its way out of every pore. But my physical discomfort was nothing compared to my longing for Jesse. I would have given anything to fast-forward my life to the point when I could once again hold him in my arms, regardless of the stinging.

Four or five hours later, we were home and reunited with our beautiful boy. He greeted us with a goofy, lopsided grin. I held him tightly and breathed in the heavenly scent of his hair. It seemed that he must have grown in the one day that we had missed. James and I exchanged glances that bundled together joy, relief, and exhaustion. It was good to be home.

Despite the painful separation from Jesse, I felt the trip had been worth it. Whether or not the banned procedure would whip my immune system into shape remained to be seen. But the greatest benefit of the trip was my comfort in the knowledge that at this moment there were at least eight other women walking around the planet with the same welts on their arms and the same scars in their hearts. I didn't wish this kind of pain on others (at least not the rational part of me, who worked tirelessly to corral the unwelcome intrusions of the bitter Stranger inside with doom fantasies for all who had the audacity to reproduce). But the encounter with my Sisters brought me immense relief. I was not alone anymore.

Chapter 22
A Match Made in Heaven

No inanimate object in my home had come to have as much instant power over my emotions as the caller ID – the anticipation at seeing James' cell phone number, the annoyance of the "Unknown" mark of a telephone solicitor, and the sheer terror at seeing the words "Santa Clara Cty." The morning in late April when those dreaded three words popped up on my caller ID, all possibilities flashed through my head. Will this be the call that finally destroys my life? Will this be the call that robs me of my son? I took a deep breath and answered. As I had suspected, Jesse's social worker, was on the other end. My heart accelerated as I steadied myself against the back of a chair.

"Hi Julie. This is Taylor. I have some news for you." Her voice betrayed nothing of the nature of the news. I resisted the urge to drop the phone and pushed myself to listen as she continued, "I have finally gotten around to contacting all of the adoptive parents of Jesse's siblings to see if they had any interest in adopting Jesse."

This was the call that I had been dreading since the day we picked up Jesse. This was the call that all of my nightmares had relentlessly played out. I was going to find out in the next instant whether or not my life was going to cease to be livable. Why did Taylor have to wait four months to finally get around to this call!! To sever my bond with Jesse at this point would be unimaginably cruel. She might as well take away sunlight or air.

I braced myself as Taylor spoke. "Julie, they all said no. So we are going to hold the matching meeting next week, and I will recommend you and James as Jesse's fost-adopt family."

Really? Was it possible that something could actually go right for James and me? Was it possible that we were going to see that irresistible chubby face gradually mature with baby teeth, permanent teeth, and even facial hair some day? Would we get the chance to hear him say his first words, see him take his first steps, hold back tears as he walked off to kindergarten? All of the scenes I had been forcing myself not to imagine fast-forwarded through my head at lightning speed. The truth I had sensed the moment the social worker unveiled his infant seat was now being affirmed. He was our son. Our son.

"Oh my God!" I spoke both to Taylor and the Big Guy Himself, "Thank you. Thank you."

The following week, we officially became Jesse's fost-adopt parents. At the matching meeting, we were enthusiastically greeted by a group of women who were over the moon with excitement about Jesse's placement with us. As they briefed us on the adoption process, Jesse flirted with each of them, making cooing noises to get their attention and then flashing his signature toothless grin. They were so charmed by him that they could barely focus on the business at hand. Nevertheless, we got through the meeting, and Jesse refrained from spitting up on himself until the very end, so it was a rousing success.

The universe was once again on our side. We were finally on the right track. Our beautiful son was on his way to being fully adopted. Our fertility problems had been identified and were being properly treated. Now we would have the best of both worlds – a successful adoption experience and a successful pregnancy. It was about time that things started going our way.

The Pursuit of Family

Chapter 23
Legends Never Die

Soon after the matching meeting, James and I had our blood redrawn at Dr. Brewer's clinic to determine whether the LIT had been effective. A couple of days later, I called the clinic, eager to hear our results. The nurse on the phone said that our results were good. What a relief – I did not want to go back to Nogales for a second round! She then said something that I was not expecting to hear.

"Did you hear that Dr. Brewer passed away yesterday?"

Come again?

"Um, no." I was not sure how to respond, "What happened?"

"He never showed up for work on Monday. We called someone to check up on him, and he was found dead in his house."

The nurse spoke with a casual tone that totally threw me off.

"Had he been sick?" I asked.

"Nothing that we thought would have killed him." She answered, "Don't worry. We will continue to run the clinic while we search for a replacement for him. Everything should continue as planned."

I was stunned by the news. Dr. Brewer was the one doctor who was able to pinpoint our problems when no one else had found a result that even bordered the edge of the normal range. He had generously handed us back the hope that had been apprehended by conventional reproductive medicine. So many people were on this earth due to Dr. Brewer. The photo albums in the lobby of the Brewer clinic displayed pictures of countless "Brewer Babies" who owe their existence to this dedicated doctor. There would be no replacing Dr. Brewer. I just hoped that the protocols that he had put in place would carry me through my next pregnancy attempt even in the absence of the man himself.

So here we were, now without our trusted doctor, jumping back on for another experience of the wild turns, glorious highs, and crushing lows of the infertility roller coaster. The particular ride we were on was more extreme than the most intimidating coaster in the Mid-Western United States, with the added feature of having an invisible track. So at any given point in time on the ride, there was never even a slight hint of what lay directly in front of us. Here James and I were again, lining up to board this stomach-turning, terror-inducing ride. As much as we hated the ride, it would be a far more terrifying option to get off of it and face life in the absence of our dream.

I had been continuing my new-found friendships with those that I had met in Nogales. We all got together practically on a daily basis on the internet board for Reproductive Immunology. The discovery of this board was another immeasurable benefit from the trip to Nogales. Out in cyberspace we gathered - people from all around the world unlucky enough to find themselves in the miniscule fraction of the population which had failed to reproduce both naturally and with the fertility treatments offered by conventional medicine. These boards freed me from my isolation. The amazing women (and some men as well) whom I found there shared their stories, knowledge, encouragement and empathy.

When given the green-light by the Brewer clinic, James and I started another Clomid cycle. This time my body didn't respond at all to the Clomid, even at the higher dose. Another delay. So we moved on to Follistim injections in the next cycle. This produced the opposite effect – my uncooperative ovaries responded too much, and I ended up with seven large follicles – way too many to be able to do an IUI. Dr. Locke was not willing to let me carry septuplets and was ready to cancel the cycle. But the rapidly pooling tears in my eyes prompted her to offer do a cyst aspiration procedure to reduce the number of follicles. In this procedure, she would insert a needle through the vaginal wall to my left ovary and inject saline into selected follicles until a reasonable number remained. A few hours and a stabbing pain later, my follicle count was down to four.

Chapter 24
Announcements

By the time of my IUI, two women I met in Nogales were already pregnant. The first was Roma, who had had three previous miscarriages. Miraculously enough, the next pregnancy announcement came from Sendy, the Indonesian woman who had been through every fertility treatment in the book, including multiple IVF cycles without ever getting pregnant. The Brewer clinic had ordered additional immune treatments for her before they would give her the green light to start an IVF cycle. She and her husband had so many issues that would prevent them from conceiving naturally that they never bothered with birth control. On the very first cycle after the LIT, they accidentally got pregnant the old fashioned way!

I was the next one in the group to announce a pregnancy. Within days of my news, Abby joined us in the pregnant group. She had been trying to conceive for years since her first miscarriage. After her LIT, she succeeded in her very first IVF cycle. I was also still keeping track of Maya, who was well into her second trimester by now. Dr. Brewer was living up to his reputation so far. I was filled with confidence that this pregnancy would be the one to go the distance.

As soon as I learned I was pregnant, I went to the Brewer clinic for blood tests to determine whether my immune system was attacking the pregnancy yet. All of the tests came back normal. My NK activation was down at six, well below the threshold of 15. Not only did this mean that my baby was safe, but it also meant that we would not have to fork over the $2500 that it cost for an IVIG treatment. At the same time, I felt a bit uneasy that maybe my problem was not my immune system after all. If my immune system had been so powerful as to kill my four other babies, why was it not acting up whatsoever with this pregnancy? While in Nogales, I had compared my numbers from the original set of blood tests with some of the other women. I found that mine were the most normal of all the ladies by far. My only number that could even raise an eyebrow, my NK activation, had been right on the border at 15. Some of the other women were up in the 30s. Was this abnormal enough to have caused four miscarriages?

At our six-week ultrasound, we breathed a sigh of relief at the glorious sight of our baby's flickering heart. The next week, we were treated to more robust heartbeats along with a healthy increase in size. At these appointments, Jesse was our lucky charm. He would flirt with all the nurses and keep us distracted as we waited. With him along, the pre-firing-squad feeling was dampened considerably. The terror was more concentrated on the ultrasound itself as opposed to being spread out over the entire waiting process. Jesse behaved perfectly during the appointments, totally unaware that the tiny little figure on the TV we were all staring at was his baby sibling.

I continued to have my blood tested to see how my immune system was reacting to the pregnancy. The morning of my eight-week ultrasound, I got a call from the Brewer clinic. Over the course of four weeks, my NK activation had jumped from a level of 6 to a whopping 17! It had crossed the safety threshold of 15, so I was going to need my first IVIG treatment. On the one hand, I was panicked that some damage had been done to my baby, but on the other hand, I was relieved to get some confirmation that we were attacking the right problem. There was no doubt now that we were on the right path. My immune system was the culprit.

Receiving the news of my NK spike piled an extra layer of stress onto an already overwhelming day. We had never had a successful eight-week ultrasound over the course of our five pregnancies. As we waited for Dr. Locke, I centered my focus on Jesse. I kept telling myself that no matter what happened today, we would still have our beautiful boy.

The ultrasound revealed that Jesse was one week closer to becoming a big brother. Everything was still normal, and we had finally passed the eight-week milestone! It was clear that the immune treatments were working.

I reported to Dr. Brewer's clinic for my first IVIG treatment the day after I heard the news of my NK spike. As the nurse at the clinic had recommended, I brought with me a packed lunch, a water bottle, and a book to pass the time during the three-hour infusion. The nurse led me to the back room of the clinic where I saw four plush recliners with soft blankets and heated pillows. To my surprise, one of the recliners was occupied by Abby, whom I had met in Nogales. Abby's body curled up casually in the recliner, with one foot tucked under her other thigh. Her face however, did not appear as relaxed as her body.

"I got the call yesterday that my NKs were at 35!" Abby said, her voice shaky, "I haven't been able to stop crying!"

Wow, that put my NK level of 17 in perspective!

"They told me not to worry – like that's possible!" Abby rolled her eyes. "This is my third IVIG treatment in the past month, and my NKs are higher than ever!"

"I'm so sorry," I responded, "I hope that this treatment brings them down finally."

There was another woman in the recliner between us who was getting a pre-conception IVIG treatment in preparation for her upcoming IVF cycle. She was very nervous about the IV, and had a mini panic attack when the infusion started. The nurse slowed down her drip and tried to calm her. Abby and I drew her into the conversation, and she relaxed a bit.

Over the course of the entire three hour infusion, my food and water vanished, but my book never saw the light of day. The three of us talked straight through, listening to each other's horror stories, empathizing as only survivors of infertility can. I found that IVIG at Dr. Brewer's clinic was more than a simple infusion of some mixed up blood product. It was a support group of sorts, albeit an insanely expensive one. Aside from the impact on my wallet, I didn't mind the treatment at all.

Ten days after my IVIG treatment, I had my blood retested to determine if my NKs had gone down. The result of this test would be a strong indicator of the ultimate outcome of the pregnancy. Some people have NKs which are completely unresponsive to IVIG, and if I fell into that category, then my baby would be defenseless against my cannibalistic immune system. If the IVIG was effective, then we would have what we needed to keep my lame-brained body in check and protect the baby.

The results were good! My NKs were down to a safe level of eight! We had dodged the bullet, and my baby was once again protected from me. For the first time in a long time, I didn't just hope for a successful pregnancy, I believed in it. My brain slowly began to release its strangle-hold on the muscles throughout my body, and my inner world softened and cooled down. Outside, the trees were greener and the flowers brighter. When the time came to pack away the tiny clothes that Jesse had outgrown, I allowed myself to linger for a moment in a vision of another small figure bringing them to life again. At one point, I even made my way to the very back of the bookcase where dusty pregnancy books had been stashed out of sight years earlier. I cracked them open again and let myself gaze at the color pictures of what my baby looked like right now.

I should have known that nothing could ever be that easy. I should have learned after being told so many times that everything was perfect, falling for it over and over like a complete dunce. Letting myself believe. How many times would I let my guard down only to have the ultrasound machine get the last laugh? I could almost hear its evil cackle leaping out of the Silence as Dr. Locke searched for my baby at my 9.5 week ultrasound.

"Is there a heartbeat?" Even though the Silence had already given me the answer, I had to ask.

"I don't have a good vision of it."

Yeah, I've heard that one before.

Unable to stall any longer, Dr. Locke gave her condolences, removed her gloves and retreated. James and I clung to Jesse and cried. Jesse seemed to sense that we were in pain. He patted our backs and snuggled with us. The love that he was able to transmit to James and me at that moment was incredibly powerful. I knew that as bad as I felt, I would never feel the same complete emptiness that I had experienced before. My intense desire for a pregnancy and a biological child had not diminished, but I knew that either way, I would survive. I knew that I was capable of being happy without realizing that dream. My family was here in my arms and out at the school where Marsha studied. My poisonous uterus would not be able to take them away.

Chapter 25
New York, New York

The Immunology Board had been buzzing for a while about Dr. Tolnai, an OBGYN and clinical pathologist based in New York. Dr. Tolnai believed that infertility and miscarriage were primarily caused by chronic, undiagnosed bacterial infections. I had seen posts on the boards about his intriguing theories, but being a one-mad-scientist-at-a-time kind of girl, I had filtered them out. With Dr. Brewer's magic lost on me, I dove head first into researching this new doctor. I desperately needed to feel like I hadn't yet exhausted all of my options. Before I even went in for the D&C, I had already read Dr. Tolnai's book and had scheduled a phone consult with him.

My research and consultation with Dr. Tolnai were enlightening. Although I had heard about STDs causing infertility, I had disregarded them as a possibility in my case because I felt there was absolutely no way for me to have gotten an STD. James had been my only sexual partner. I was his second, but his first had been a virgin. Plus, I felt like I would have had some symptoms of infection if I had one, or at least the screenings at my annual physicals would have detected it. But what I learned from Dr. Tolnai is that some chronic infections which affect fertility can be passed down through the generations. Many people carry these infections and are completely unaware. Conventional tests typically do not detect the chronic forms of these bacteria. Oftentimes, the carriers of the infections don't even have issues with fertility. But Dr. Tolnai believes that there can be signs of the infection in their babies such as allergies, asthma, and chronic health issues stemming from immune system overload. It is only when an infection meets a vigorous immune system that fertility problems arise.

The way Dr. Tolnai described it, the infection lives in your body, pretty much unnoticed. It creates an environment which is hostile toward pregnancy. If pregnancy occurs, the immune system shuts down in the pelvis, as it is supposed to, to prevent itself from attacking the baby. This halting of the immune system gives the infection license to populate the uterus. At some point, a vigilant immune system has to take notice, and it turns itself back on, attacking both the infection and the developing fetus.

Going over my history, Dr. Tolnai was able to point out a few clear signs of infection. Before I was married, my cycles had been around 30 days. After going off the pill, they were more like 35 days. Then with each cycle, they increasingly lengthened, until they reached the excruciating *40 days and 40 nights in the desert* that they were at this point. Dr. Tolnai explained that infection commonly causes lengthening, shortening and otherwise disruption of the natural cycle.

Also after my first pregnancy, I had that stubborn case of bacterial vaginosis which took three rounds of antibiotics to resolve. Bacterial vaginosis is conventionally thought of as a disproportionate population of "good" bacteria, or bacteria that is a normal part of the vaginal flora. However, Dr. Tolnai asserted that the root cause of this imbalance is usually a "bad" bacteria, which has no business being in the reproductive system. Tests which conventional doctors run for bacterial vaginosis only conclude that there is an overgrowth of bacteria. They do not identify the specific bacteria responsible. Dr. Tolnai noted that the series of antibiotics I took not only cleared up the bacterial vaginosis, but also cleared up the "bad" bacteria enough that I was able to achieve that seemingly miraculous "first-try" pregnancy. Out of the five pregnancies thus far, there was only one other that was not helped along by IUI, and that one took nine months to establish. Although the antibiotics helped me to get pregnant, they were evidently not able to entirely clear my reproductive system of "bad" bacteria. The buggers repopulated and ultimately caused the pregnancy to end with same disastrous outcome.

Dr. Tolnai's course of treatment required a ten day stay in New York for daily antibiotic treatments for both the husband and the wife. The cost of the testing and treatment came to a grand total of $12,000. However, due to the diagnosis of Pelvic Inflammatory Disease rather than Infertility, many people were able to get their insurance to cover at least some portion of it. At this point, I literally didn't care what it cost. This sounded like it was the answer that we had been looking for which would finally lead us to a successful pregnancy. Besides, the thought of having bacterial invaders milling about inside of us gave me the willies. I wanted those bugs gone ASAP!

We boarded a plane to New York in mid-September. This time, since we were not leaving the country, there was nothing that could keep us from taking our now eight-month old Jesse along. We hoped that perhaps the time spent outside of the doctor's office could be a mini vacation for the three of us. Luckily, we had been able to get both the plane tickets using credit card miles, and my extremely loving parents, grandmother, aunt and uncle all chipped in to pay for our hotel room. This helped slow the traffic out of what had become a revolving-door entrance to our savings account.

We stayed in a hotel in a nice part of Central Park West. The clinic was in Central Park East, so getting there required a daily walk through the park. Thus far, I had only seen Central Park on film, but I instantly discovered that an in-person view of it is really the only way to do it justice. The rolling hills, the shimmering bodies of water, the charming horse-drawn carriages - this place was a seemingly endless, grassy wonderland. It had a hypnotic impact on me, reversing the effect of the crowded bustle of the city whose skyline jutted out along the perimeter.

However, James and I grossly underestimated the immensity and complexity of the park. Getting to the other side wasn't just a simple case of walking in a vaguely easterly direction. The paths twisted and turned. Our first day there, we got completely disoriented and spent a large block of time wandering in circles until we finally popped back out into the city. A sense of direction was not something that either James or I were capable of genetically bestowing upon a biological child. With us as parents, our baby would be lucky to find his or her way out of the birth canal. Miraculously, a look at the *E* printed on the street signs told us that we had somehow managed to make it to the eastern side. Thankful that the streets in New York are conveniently arranged in numerical order, we were able to find our way to Dr. Tolnai's office, arriving with a bit of time to spare before our appointment.

We sat on couches in Dr. Tolnai's waiting room, listening for the nurse to call us to the office. To our surprise, Dr. Tolnai himself came out to greet us, his expansive personality immediately filling the room. He cheerfully shook our hands and led us to his office. Once seated, he reviewed with us our long and sordid pregnancy history. Somehow even in the midst of such a complete downer of a topic, Dr. Tolnai managed to keep the mood light, artfully balancing between sympathy and humor that bordered on teasing.

The next step was the testing. Dr. Tolnai didn't waste any time as he irreverently grabbed a swab from James' urethra – that was a tight squeeze for a Q-tip! James donated another sperm sample, and we both whipped out our arms again for more blood-letting. Poor James took one for the team as he underwent an ultrasound examination of his prostate, the wand of the ultrasound machine navigating its way up the only wand-accessible hole on a man (use your imagination). Dr. Tolnai noted that there was some scarring in James' prostate. It was not severe, but significant enough to be a sign of infection.

I was next in line for invasive procedures. I endured another ultrasound examination of my pelvis which appeared normal. Next Dr. Tolnai took a vaginal and cervical swab. To obtain a sample of the uterine lining, Dr. Tolnai performed an endometrial biopsy. This was my second experience of this procedure and by far the least painful. I only felt slight cramping as he skillfully snatched the sample.

The results of the tests would be trickling in over the next few weeks. James and I agreed to undergo the therapy without yet receiving the test results. We didn't want to take two trips to New York. Also, there was a chance that the tests could come back with a false negative. So we wanted to be safe and get the treatment based on our empirical symptoms which according to Dr. Tolnai, strongly indicated infection.

Dr. Tolnai and his nurse worked together to thread IVs into the arms of both James and me. Each IV was hooked up to an ambulatory pump which would deliver a cocktail of antibiotics over the next ten days. The mix of medicine was designed to eliminate a broad range of the most common bacterial offenders. The pump was housed in a small black fanny pack – hello 1980's! Fashion faux pas aside, the IV was not terribly uncomfortable.

However the word "uncomfortable" would understate James' next experience to the point of insult. He received his first of the five prostate shots which he would be repeating every other day over the course of our stay. The nightmarish shots were delivered, guided by the aforementioned ultrasound wand, probing once again into the aforementioned hole. The ultrasound helped Dr. Tolnai to aim the needle, which was hydraulically triggered, piercing through the anal wall straight into the prostate. James received no anesthesia, and man, he could have used it! No one could say that he wasn't taking his fair share of the physical pain.

Poor James, the color completely drained from his face, tenderly sat back on the waiting room couch to recover from the insult to his insides. Jesse, exhausted from the plane ride, peacefully slept in the stroller by his side, unaware of the entire ordeal.

It was my turn to face my fate for the ensuing days as I received my first of ten uterine lavages. In this procedure, Dr. Tolnai threaded a catheter directly into my uterus. Antibiotics were pumped in through the catheter and my uterus was literally bathed in the medicine for about 45 minutes. I would not describe this as one of the most painful procedures that I have had. Basically I felt a cramp when the catheter was inserted. During the wash itself, there was no pain. It was uncomfortable to sit with legs up in the stirrups for 45 minutes. My feet were asleep after the first 20. But I did get to read several novels over the course of the treatment, so I couldn't complain too much, especially given the extreme suffering my husband was enduring in the next room.

And so continued our daily ritual in New York. Continental hotel breakfast, peaceful stroll through Central Park, treatments at Dr. Tolnai's office, sack lunch of peanut butter and jelly, lots of aimless walking around the city. Wanting to pack light, we had not brought Jesse's car seat, and we were too intimidated to tackle the subway system with a baby and a stroller. So the only places we visited were walking-distance attractions. Luckily, in NYC, there are attractions pretty much everywhere.

Our first tourist visit was the Natural History Museum. Jesse didn't care much about the displays, but he had a grand time at the museum. Having recently figured out how fun it was to say "Ba ba ba ba," he was endlessly delighted by the echo effect created by his booming voice and the acoustics of the space.

Not in the mindset for the city pace, we spent most of our time in Central Park, visiting the zoo and various playgrounds. Since Jesse was not crawling yet, there was not much that he could really do at a park. But he enjoyed swinging and watching the other children.

Aside from the fact that he did not sleep at night for more than an hour or two at a time during the trip, Jesse was a model traveler. His precious babble, goofy grin, and incredibly squeezable thighs had the power to instantly wipe clean our memory of why we were on this trip.

However, at times it was impossible to forget why we were there. James was the most tortured by the treatments. By the third night, he started waking with fevers and chills. Dr. Tolnai explained that these were "die-off" symptoms caused by a large load of bacteria dying at once, releasing toxins throughout the body. Both of us were exhausted from the journey, the treatments, and a sleepless baby. The metallic taste of antibiotic, a side effect of the IV, lingered in our mouths, dampening our enjoyment of the local cuisine. We were a dangerous combination - two haggard, sleep-deprived people with only one another for adult company. By the eighth day, bickering had overtaken a large portion of our interactions.

On the ninth day, we were granted a furlough from our misery. Father Gilbert, the priest who had married us, happened to be in New York. We had dinner and took a long evening walk with him. I don't believe that Catholic priests have any special powers by virtue of being priests. In fact, I would rate many of the priests over my three decades of Catholicism as being some of the last sources that I would tap for understanding and wisdom regarding my life. But there was something magical about Father Gilbert's presence. He made us laugh and transported us back to the happier times. As confused as I was about God and how to place religion in light of my experiences, being in the presence of Father Gilbert made me certain that there was a deeper meaning beyond our day-to-day existence. It was not because he preached to us at all, because the encounter was more like old friends catching up. There was just something intangible that he transmitted which calmed me from the inside out. As we walked back to our New York home, James and I were transformed. I made a note to myself that this feeling is what I want to conjure when I wrestle with my brain's image of God.

Chapter 26
There's No Place like Home

There's nothing that makes you appreciate home quite like staying for ten days in a cramped hotel, washing baby bottles in a bathroom sink for a baby who has given up nighttime sleeping. After our plane landed, I felt like dropping down on all fours and kissing the warm, golden California ground.

A couple of weeks after arriving home, we received our test results from Dr. Tolnai's office. They confirmed what Dr. Tolnai had suspected. My vaginal, cervical, and endometrial swabs all came up positive for significant overgrowth of bacteria typically native to the vagina. James as well turned up positive for several overgrowths of native bacteria and one particular bacteria which had no business whatsoever in the reproductive tract. Dr. Tolnai believed that this "bad" bacteria was the cause of all of our problems and that even though I tested negative for it, we had to assume that I had it as well. We just had to hope that the aggressive treatments we received had wiped out every last bugger. With the results, Dr. Tolnai instructed us to wait two months to allow our systems to get back to normal before trying for another pregnancy. November could not come soon enough.

October came with the pleasant surprise of a 29 day menstrual cycle! This was a strong indication that the treatments had done their job and had normalized my system.

Another October surprise was that Jesse started walking. He had been determined to walk for quite some time, and finally worked out the kinks at a mere 9 ½ months of age. However, there was something odd about his stiff little gait. And each time he lost his balance, he would further stiffen and plummet in a backwards swan dive, landing directly on his head. He also wasn't crawling yet. He had recently worked out a wounded-soldier type creeping motion that allowed him some mobility on the floor, but it was a far cry from a proper crawl. His pediatrician reassured me that he was normal, but I'd seen early walkers with their signature bottom-plopping falls. Babies are as sure to land on their bottoms as cats are on their feet. This was not normal.

Based upon the advice of a Public Health Nurse, I asked Jesse's pediatrician to refer him to the Early Start program so that he could be evaluated. The Early Start team did a thorough evaluation of Jesse's vision, hearing, language, motor skills, social skills, and cognitive development. In every area except for gross motor skills, Jesse was average or well above average. It was reassuring to see formal proof of how well he was doing. However, in gross motor skills, he was significantly behind. Despite the fact that he was walking, he had missed many of the milestones that were supposed to come first. And his walking was clearly dangerous. I had become a full-time spotter, following him around all day to prevent him from smashing his skull on the ground. The Early Start team concluded that Jesse qualified to receive one hour per week of physical therapy.

On her first visit, the physical therapist observed Jesse for only a few minutes and was able to notice many subtle things about his movement that an untrained eye would never notice. He pulled himself up to a stand by planting both feet on the floor and shooting his body upright, rather than standing from a half-kneel (one knee and one foot on the floor). He was unable to transition directly from a seated position to a crawling position. He was unable to maintain a seated position for long periods of time. When he would pick things up off of the floor from a standing position, he would only bend at the waist. To remedy these problems, one thing she advised us to do was to push his hips down, forcing him into a squatting position as often as possible. This would get his body more comfortable with bending. Also, she found that Jesse was missing certain key reflexes. When he fell forward or backward, he didn't put his hands out to catch his fall. To correct this problem, we had to repeatedly hurl his little body toward the floor and train him to put his arms out to catch himself. It felt very contrary to basic parental instinct to do this, but it actually worked. We immediately started seeing improvements after the start of the therapy sessions. I was so glad that we had the help we needed to address these problems while he was still very young so they wouldn't become larger problems later.

Chapter 27
Pain Relief

When November finally arrived, and we were one week away from starting afresh with an infection-free try for pregnancy, I suddenly came down with what seemed to be a urinary tract infection. I had discomfort in my bladder that made it feel completely full no matter how many times I tried to empty it. I called Dr. Tolnai, and he said that it was probably a simple e coli infection. I went to the local doctor for a culture, and it came back negative. Thinking the test was incorrect, Dr. Tolnai put me on antibiotics anyway. Still the bladder discomfort continued. I couldn't sleep at night. I started spending my nights on the couch, pillows propping me semi-upright, watching television to distract from the pain until I would eventually drift off to sleep.

Desperate for an expert opinion, I visited a local urologist. Without examining me or testing me for anything, he wrote me a prescription for Detrol, suggesting that I take it for the rest of my life. Recognizing Detrol as the drug featured in the "Gotta go, gotta go, gotta go!" TV adds, featuring menopausal women with incontinence issues, I quickly concluded that this man was not to be trusted. I ran from that office, and never looked back.

I got my NK's tested at Dr. Brewer's clinic, and they were through the roof – higher than they had ever been! I didn't know if that indicated an infection or just that my immune system was hyped up for some reason. Dr. Tolnai continued to insist that it was an infection, and all local doctors consistently and vehemently discredited Dr. Tolnai. My brain cells darted aimlessly through space, like a flock of agitated birds before a storm. This was a new low for me. Not only did I not have a biological baby, but now I had a chronic health problem. Did my stubborn quest for a baby put me in this state? Was my health permanently damaged by one of the treatments I had subjected my body to as I pushed it to accept the baby it didn't want me to have? Was chronic pain going to be the new norm for me?

I continued like this for months, desperately searching the internet, pleading for advice on the boards. Some suggested that the culprit might be yeast because of all of the antibiotics I had taken in New York. I looked into dietary changes I could make to minimize yeast. I completely cut out all simple sugars from my diet, only eating fresh, natural, whole ingredients. Still no improvement.

Next, I came across a nurse on the East Coast who was a survivor of this mysterious bladder pain, sometimes referred to as interstitial cystitis. She now had her own practice devoted to helping people with bladder pain. I contacted her, and submitted to a series of tests, including sending my pee off in the mail to be analyzed using a broth culture. This type of culture was supposedly better at identifying infections than testing done in local labs. The results of the first culture showed an enterococcus infection. So I went on antibiotics to battle the enterococcus. Still, I felt no relief. The next time I sent my urine off, it came back with a completely different bacterial infection for which I took more antibiotics. And it continued like this for at least three more cultures, each discovering some new infection, but nothing putting any dent in my symptoms. The nurse told me that there were multiple layers of infection in my bladder, and we just had to get down to the bottom layer. By March, this nurse had decided that I had Lyme Disease, and told me that I needed to go on heavy antibiotics for a year to treat the disease. How could I possibly have Lyme Disease? I'd only been to the East Coast once in my life for my ten days with Dr. Tolnai. I had never even seen a tick, much less been bitten by one. Really, what were the odds? I knew I was cursed, but come on, as generally healthy as I was, how many rare, serious chronic infections could I possibly have? I felt more hopeless than ever.

Over these long months, there was one medicine that had worked to bring temporary relief to my bladder pain, and his name was Jesse. With a delightful little toddler around, my focus could not linger for long on pain. My bladder wasn't even on the radar on June 27, 2007. This was the day that the county of Santa Clara officially recognized what I had known since the first day I had laid eyes on my little miracle. On that day, almost 18 months after that fateful, winter night, James and I brought our boy to the courthouse for his adoption hearing.

For his court appearance, Jesse wore cute little khaki slacks with a long sleeve shirt and sweater vest. He looked like a perfect little gentleman. When we entered the courtroom, there was a huge stack of stuffed animals from which Jesse could take his pick. He test-hugged each one, and finally settled on a little tan monkey.

The judge, smiling and friendly, reviewed with us our rights and responsibilities as Jesse's legal parents. We raised our right hands and swore to fulfill our obligation to Jesse. We signed all the documents and watched the judge sign. Then it was over. After some picture taking, we left the court house as Jesse's official, legal, forever parents. This was the moment that I had been fantasizing about for 18 months. Altogether, the whole process took less than 15 minutes. To me, the occasion deserved a parade, or at least a trumpet fanfare. In reality it was anticlimactic. I kept checking myself to see if I felt different now that things were official, like I did after the moment I said my vows on my wedding day. But I realized that nothing had actually changed in my relationship with Jesse like it had when my fiancé became my husband. Jesse had always been my son. Now it was just legally binding. But I did know for sure that it would be an enormous weight off of my mind to know that no one would be swooping down and taking my son away from me. He was stuck with us for good! Thank God!

Chapter 28
What Goes Up Must Come Down and Up and Down Again

Although I wasn't about to go through a year's worth of Lyme Disease treatment, I did need to do something about my bladder. I finally decided to listen to Dr. Tolnai and come back to New York for additional treatments. This time, I would have another IV, plus uterine and bladder lavages. I traveled by myself in July for five days of treatments. After I returned home, I started feeling like my body had lost its mind. Sudden attacks of high fevers repeatedly appeared and vanished, leaving me a sweaty, achy mess for a full two weeks. I wondered if these were bacterial die-off symptoms, like James had experienced in New York. When the fevers resolved, I noticed slight improvement in my bladder. As the weeks went by, the trend continued. Some days, I didn't even notice my bladder. By September, I was mostly pain free, having one or two bad days, here or there. My NK count finally settled down. Exactly one year after our initial trip to see Dr. Tolnai, we were finally ready to try for a pregnancy.

My cycles were still at a nice 29 day length, so I figured we had a much better shot at a natural pregnancy. We opted to also do preconception IVIG just to make sure that my immune system was in check. This was an expensive option, but I didn't want my NK's spiking in the early weeks of pregnancy like they did the last time.

Not wanting to leave anything to chance, I also got the paperwork started for a second adoption home study. If we had another failed pregnancy, I wanted everything in place to do a second adoption. I wanted Jesse to grow up with a sibling close to his age.

One sunny day in late September, I spontaneously decided to take Jesse to Happy Hollow, a local park and zoo. It was a perfect day at the park - just what I needed to get my mind in a positive mode for our next try at pregnancy. As I was loading Jesse in the car to return home, my cell phone rang. The screen displayed the name of Jesse's social worker. My heart immediately started turning somersaults. Had something gone wrong with the adoption? Was he going to be taken away from me after all?

I tentatively answered, and when Christine greeted me, she sounded completely deflated. Something had happened. My body made the sudden transition from peaceful park mode to five-alarm mode.

"Hi Julie. I'm calling because I just got a call from Fresno County Social Services. Apparently Graciana (Jesse's birth mother) is at it again. She has just given birth to a baby girl. I was wondering if you and James had any interest."

I had been pushed out of the way of the speeding bus only to be trampled by a stampede of elephants. Thankfully, Jesse was still secure as my son, but this unexpected news knocked me right off my feet. *A new baby now*? We already had a 20 month old baby who, although fantastically delightful, was a heck of a lot of work. We had a 16 year old, who was on the brink of important milestones and life decisions, deserving our attention and guidance. We were just about to try to get pregnant and face a whole new set of challenges. How could we possibly bring a newborn into the picture with all that we were already dealing with, much less one who was drug-exposed and would likely have the same, if not worse, issues that we were facing with Jesse?

At the same time, this was Jesse's sister. How could we keep him separate from his sister? The second I allowed the possibility to creep in, my mind was flooded with images of another warm, snuggly infant with a similar DNA makeup to our heavenly boy. It was a wildly tantalizing picture.

Snapping back to reality, I realized I needed to respond to Christine. "Umm, what do you know about her?" That's right, if James were here, he would be asking before leaping.

"Well, she was born four days ago. She was healthy, but tested positive for meth, so Fresno County placed her in emergency foster care. She weighed 6 lbs, 8 oz. Her name is Natalie."

A couple of pregnancies ago, my belief in signs from on high had retreated to the place in my mind where I keep unicorns and leprechauns. But my ears had heard it. Out of the entire universe of names, this baby, Jesse's sister, had the one name that James and I had chosen for our baby girl long before we were even married. Natalie was not a strange name, but not particularly common either. What were the odds? Out of the corner of my eye, I could swear I spotted a winged, white mammal soaring across the sky. If this wasn't meant to be, then what was?

"I will talk to James about it," I responded to Christine, "But I'm pretty sure that we are interested."

James and I talked through the possibility of adopting Natalie. As usual, he was more cautious than I, but came to the same conclusion that he wanted Natalie to join our family, regardless of the risk. I phoned Christine and let her know our decision. She would call the social worker in Fresno and set the wheels in motion for us.

Days passed, and we never heard from Christine or anyone in Fresno. I left multiple messages with Christine and never heard back. Precious time that we could be spending bonding with Natalie was slipping away.

Finally I caught Christine in the office. She apologized for not getting back to me, but said that she had left multiple messages for Natalie's worker in Fresno that had not been returned. She gave me the number of Natalie's social worker so that I could try phoning as well. After several days of calling every hour or so and leaving multiple voice messages, someone finally picked up the phone. I explained to the voice on the other end the reason for my call.

"Well," the woman responded, "We are currently in the process of looking for placement for Natalie. There are several relatives on her father's side who are interested in adopting her. However, we cannot evaluate them until we confirm through DNA testing that the alleged father is the actual father. He has submitted his blood for testing."

The father had not even entered my mind! Of course Natalie had a different father from Jesse with a different set of relatives. Jesse's father had never been found to DNA test, so he had never been an issue. Apparently this was not the case with Natalie's father. And I knew from Pride class that blood relatives always get first priority. But what about Jesse? Arguably, he was her closest blood relative. Didn't he count for something?

I proceeded to question the worker, "So if this man turns out to be Natalie's biological father, then would all of these relatives have priority over me, even though her closest sibling lives with me?"

"That is correct." She responded matter-of-factly. "However, if you would like us to place her with you in the meantime as a concurrent placement, then we can do that."

I imagined bringing Natalie home and falling for her in the same instantaneous way that I fell for Jesse. We would explain to Jesse that this was his sister, and he would fall in love as well. Then a few short weeks later, she would be ripped out of our lives. That did not make sense for us or for Natalie. I spoke to James about it as well, and we both agreed to wait for the paternity test results rather than have Natalie placed with us.

Every week, I called the social worker and left messages asking if the paternity test results had come back. Every week, I got no response. In the meantime, we had two tries for a natural pregnancy, both of which failed, flushing another $5k down the proverbial tubes. At that point, we decided to get reacquainted with our trusty old friend IUI. Our first attempt failed and another $2500 slipped out of our pockets.

Finally, a full two months after Natalie's birth, I received a call back from her social worker.

"The DNA results have come in." Natalie's worker said. I braced myself to hear the results which would finally shut the door on our hopes of taking Natalie home. The results which would forever lock away in my mind any possibility that there was any spark of the Divine reaching down into our lives on earth. As she spoke, I could hear the click of the door handle, the turning of the dead bolt, "It turns out that the alleged father is in fact not the biological father."

The rays of the sun suddenly burst through the passageways in my mind. "Really," I said as the blood started pumping its way to my numb extremities, "Does that mean that we can take her home?"

"Well, there's actually one relative on the mother's side who we need to evaluate. But if she does not qualify, then you would be next in line."

WHAT!! Ok, do I have some sort of sign on my back that says "Jerk me around!"? Do the prevailing powers in the universe have some ongoing bet as to how many times we can raise and dash Julie's hopes before she goes completely bonkers? How did they turn someone up on the mother's side after 11 other babies had been born and all adopted or fostered out?

"How long will it take to evaluate this relative?" I asked.

"Several weeks," the social worker responded.

I asked one more time for clarification, "So basically if it turns out that this person is not a criminal, then we have no chance of getting Natalie. Is that right?"

"Yes," she responded, "That is how it works."

So I told Natalie's social worker that we would wait for this woman to be evaluated, and that we did not want to take Natalie home in the meantime. I wanted to hurl the phone across the room.

As I calmed down from my initial reaction to the news about Natalie, I gradually came to the conclusion that it was all for the best. It just didn't make sense to add a high-risk infant to our already full plates. As Jesse got closer to turning two, it was becoming clear that speech was very difficult for him. At this point, he was seeing a speech therapist, an occupational therapist, and an early interventionist, all on a weekly basis. The speech therapist had recently diagnosed him with dyspraxia, a neurological problem that impacts overall motor planning. This diagnosis explained some of his physical delays as well as his speech difficulties. I could see how impossible it would be to raise two children with issues, juggling all of their therapy appointments, and working with them both at home. Yes, it was for the best that she would be going to someone else. But why did her name have to be Natalie? It just seemed so cruel that on top of losing a baby girl for us and a sister for Jesse, we had also lost the name itself. We couldn't very well name another sister of Jesse's Natalie now that he already had one.

We went back to Stanford for a second IUI attempt in December. On the day of our IUI, I got a call from Natalie's social worker informing me that the mom's relative had passed the evaluation. It was finished. Natalie was not going to be ours. Even though I knew that this was the most likely outcome, I had still been holding out a small glimmer of hope that it would somehow go the other way. I felt the loss sharply and deeply. But James and I gave each other a quick pep talk about how it was all for the best, and after re-enumerating the multitude of reasons, we were both almost convinced.

Two weeks following our IUI, James and I were stunned by yet another negative pregnancy test. Not only were we not getting Natalie, but we were not getting pregnant.

One December morning, as my mother and I stood in my kitchen baking Christmas cookies, I got a call from Kim, Jesse's former court-appointed child advocate. If there is such a thing a living saint, Kim is one of them. Kim had been assigned to Jesse when he was a foster child because she was also the child advocate for Jesse's two teenaged brothers who were in long-term foster care. Her work with Jesse's brothers was a volunteer position that she did on top of her very busy job as a photographer. She was a constant source of support and guidance for the boys. She facilitated visits between Jesse and all four of the siblings who were in the area. She was actively searching for the other six siblings whom we hadn't yet met. Kim had helped us immensely by pushing the court to speed up Jesse's adoption process. Without her, it would have taken even longer than the seemingly endless 18 months.

On the phone, Kim sounded breathless, like she couldn't get the words from her brain to my ears fast enough.

"Julie, I've been thinking so much about Natalie. The way this has been going just seemed so wrong to me. So I called Fresno and found out who Natalie's DA is."

Woah, hang on a sec! We have closed the book on that one more times than I can count. I do not want to go there again.

But Kim went on.

"So yesterday, I finally spoke to Polly, Natalie's DA, and she was shocked to hear about you guys. Apparently, Natalie's social worker barely even mentioned you in her report, only saying that you weren't interested in Natalie being placed with you. So I was like, 'She's been calling the social worker once a week. Is that how people act when they're not interested?' Anyway, I told Polly that I wanted the kids to be able to have contact with each other. The family that they're placing Natalie with lives way down south on the border of San Diego and Mexico. The woman is a very, very distant cousin of Graciana. It doesn't make sense to place Natalie there with some obscure relative when so many of her family members are here in the Bay Area, including her closest brother. I told her that Natalie should be placed with you." Kim paused for a second and then could not contain her excitement. "And she agreed!"

I hesitated to process this information. Having spent the past month or so actively convincing myself that it was for the best that Natalie be placed elsewhere, I would have a lot of self-brainwashing to undo before I could fully embrace this idea. Plus, I was not eager for another round of Charlie Brown and Lucy football antics. I knew from bitter experience that every time I let my guard down and trusted in an outcome, I always ended up with my hind end slammed squarely on the unforgiving ground.

Skepticism in hand, I questioned Kim further, "Who has more power, the DA or the social worker?"

Kim said, "I'm not really sure, but I believe that if they don't agree with each other, then the final decision comes down to the judge."

I thanked Kim profusely for her intervention on our behalf, though I still wasn't certain how I felt about it. My head spun round on its seemingly permanent yo-yo string. Of course I still had a deep yearning to bring that baby girl home. But even with the DA in our corner it could still go either way. How many times could I lose Natalie before enough was enough?

I could tell right away that Polly, Natalie's DA, was someone who made things happen, even in the snail-slow system of social services. The very next day, I got a call from Natalie's social worker saying that the DA wanted her to evaluate our family. She asked me a series of questions regarding our family. In the meantime, Polly recommended that Kim and I both write letters to the judge explaining why Natalie would be best placed in our home.

As we awaited a decision regarding Natalie, we did not put the brakes on our pregnancy attempts. We had another failed IUI in late January. In each of the five attempts we had made since my bladder had recovered, we had coughed up $2500 for preconception IVIG, not to mention all of the copayments for multiple ultrasounds. The IUI procedure itself was also not covered by insurance, and cost us around $400 each time. I started crunching numbers and came to the conclusion that it may be ultimately cheaper to move to the more expensive in-vitro fertilization (IVF) and have it work in one try rather than repeating IUI attempts indefinitely. Also my wild ovaries were tough to control with IUI because at one dose they would produce nothing, but at the next higher dose, they would produce way too many, putting us at high risk for multiples. This kind of ovary, however, was perfect for IVF in which you want as many mature follicles as possible so that you have more eggs to fertilize. The more embryos the better because then you can pick the very best ones to transfer back.

So I shopped around for the best IVF clinic for the money and settled on Zoumis Fertility Center in Daly City.

Many of my friends from the reproductive immunology boards had been very successful with Dr. Zoumis. I also had had several IVIG buddies who had raved about what a great doctor he was. So I mentally prepared myself to start this new process after one cycle of wait. I figured that at this point, I would have had every fertility treatment known to humankind.

Natalie's hearing took place in late February, and that afternoon, Polly called me with the news that our family had been chosen as Natalie's fost-adopt placement. I literally jumped up and down and danced around my family room after hanging up the phone. As much protection as I had placed in front of my heart, the bottom line was that from the moment I heard of Natalie's existence, I had been aching to be her mother.

Chapter 29
A Face in the Distance

As the news about Natalie settled into my consciousness, I found it very surreal to think about this five month old girl living two hours from our home. I had never met her and didn't know anything about her other than her name. Yet she was my daughter. Was she crying right at this very moment? Was she in a home with people who loved her and took good care of her? And if so, how would she feel about us ripping her away from the only family she'd ever known? I just hoped that we would be able to take her home soon so that we wouldn't lose any more precious bonding time or miss any more baby milestones.

Of course nothing could just go smoothly. Following the Wednesday hearing, Natalie's social worker was supposed to call me to set up the transition. But the phone never rang. On Monday, I started calling every ten or so minutes to catch the worker in her office, and after several hours of trying, I finally made contact. My heart sunk as the worker explained the process to me. First, a transition meeting would have to take place with our family, the social worker, and the foster family. That could not be scheduled until the following week because the social worker had no open slots in her schedule. Once that meeting had occurred, then the foster family would have to be given a seven day notice. At the end of the waiting period, we could finally take Natalie home. This added up to at least two more weeks of wait! I asked if at the very least, the social worker could give my phone number to the foster mom so that I could make contact with her and possibly schedule a visit with Natalie. That way, at least James and I could start getting to know our daughter even if the weighty process was preventing us from taking her home. The social worker agreed.

Two days later, Natalie's foster mother called. I was eager, but quite apprehensive to speak with Melissa. It's not an everyday occurrence to speak to the woman who has been raising your child since birth. I had compiled a long list of questions to ask her regarding Natalie's likes and dislikes, her schedule, her personality. Melissa answered every single question in great detail, clearly demonstrating that she knew Natalie inside and out. When she spoke of Natalie, her voice carried a smile across the phone lines. In fact, she revealed that she wanted to adopt Natalie as well. It struck me that she was in the exact same position that I had been in as Jesse's emergency foster mother. Only in her case, there *was* someone with more priority who wanted Natalie. I felt very guilty being that person. But Melissa seemed resigned to the fact that Natalie was going to be placed with biological family. If it wasn't our family, then it would have been the cousin anyway. I asked her if she could email me a picture, and she agreed, adding that she had a whole cd of pictures of Natalie to give me when we came to pick her up. Melissa wanted the transition to be smooth and offered to waive the seven day notice so that Natalie could come home and start bonding with us sooner. I was so impressed by her clear focus on Natalie's best interest. I wondered if I could have been so selfless had the roles been reversed.

After hanging up with Melissa, I checked my inbox every few minutes, looking for the pictures of Natalie that she had promised. I couldn't wait to see what she looked like. Would she strongly resemble Jesse? Would seeing her face help me to connect with her as my child?

When the pictures finally arrived, I was so excited that I could barely coordinate my hands to get the mouse to double click. When I opened the first one, I breathlessly watched as the first glimpse of my baby daughter appeared on the screen. She was a strikingly beautiful little girl, with a lush mop of black hair, pulled haphazardly into many small pony tails. Her face was quite similar to Jesse's, yet her eyes were more almond-shaped with prominent eyebrows. She had a distinctively native look to her, like a gorgeous little Mayan princess. Even though she was a very petite girl, her long hair made her appear much older than five months. This was a harsh reminder to me of all of the baby time that we had missed with her. As each minute slipped by, how much was she growing and changing?

Even though I wouldn't feel 100% sure that Natalie was really coming home with us until we had her strapped into our car, I knew that some preparations could not wait for that moment. James and I got books and DVDs for Jesse which featured little boys getting new baby siblings. Not having the luxury of nine months of preparation nor the physical evidence of a growing belly to help him understand, he would need a crash course. Even if he were able to mentally comprehend what was about to happen, I wasn't sure how he would handle losing his only-baby status. As it was at this point, Jesse's world fell apart any time he saw me holding another baby. I worried about how he would respond to his sudden sibling. When we read the books to him, it was clear that he didn't grasp the parallel between himself and the boys in the stories who were getting baby sisters. It wasn't until we set up Natalie's crib that he started conceptualizing the fact that there was going to be a new little tenant in our house. When we asked him who was going to sleep in the crib, his grin would broaden as he said, "Baby Nah Nah." I hoped that he would still be grinning after the little intruder's arrival.

A couple of days after I had spoken to Melissa, Natalie's DA called me asking if we had brought Natalie home yet. I filled her in on the long process that the social worker had laid out for transitioning Natalie. With an exasperated sigh, Polly explained to me that in cases like this, where everyone is in agreement, there is no need for a transition meeting, nor for seven day notice. She reassured me that she would call the social worker's supervisor and straighten things out.

Sure enough, Natalie's social worker called back, saying that we could skip all of the formalities and pick

Natalie up the following Wednesday. At long last, our baby girl was coming home!

On March 5, 2008, James and I made our way to Fresno to bring our Natalie home. Outside of the car, the world was in an unusually peaceful state. Traffic flowed with the smoothness of a bird migration. The gentle morning sunlight reflected upon the almost fluorescent green of the hills, hinting at the imminence of springtime. The San Luis reservoir glistened without a ripple in sight.

My awe at the outside world was in direct contrast to the tossing and turning of my inner world. I was eager to meet Natalie and bring her home, but my fears regarding my ability to handle this new responsibility had not subsided. Melissa had indicated that Natalie did not show severe effects of the drugs, but she did mention that Natalie awakened every 2-3 hours during the night. And during the long nights at our house, she would undoubtedly be crying for the Mommy that she had known since her birth. Would she be angry at us for stealing her from Melissa? To add to my disquiet, I was still wrestling with the lurking fear that something would go wrong in Fresno and we would not end up taking her home today.

All of these thoughts were thrashing about my mind when we arrived at Melissa's home. James and I looked at each other and took a deep breath. This was it. Jesse's baby sister, our daughter, was on the other side of that door.

Moments after we knocked, the door flew open. We were greeted by the adorable, dimpled smile of Melissa's three year old son Jack Jr. He was overjoyed to see that we had brought a gift to thank him for being a good foster brother to Natalie. I wondered if he comprehended that he would be losing his baby sister to another little boy today. Standing behind Jack Jr, Melissa warmly ushered us into her living room. In the corner, an infant swing rocked back and forth, cradling a very small figure with thick, dark hair drawn up like a palm tree on the top of her head. Melissa scooped up the tiny child and brought her toward us.

"This is Natalie," Melissa said as she held the baby facing outward.

Catching sight of the interesting strangers, Natalie's face exploded into an open-mouth, toothless smile, reminiscent of a gleeful Muppet. She engaged with us immediately, communicating a playful exuberance that had not been captured in the pictures that Melissa had sent. Melissa immediately handed her to me. She was so lightweight that if not for her squirming and wriggling, I would barely notice that I was holding anything. James and I played with her, making faces and shaking rattles. Giggling, she batted at the rattles. This was promising. She was happy and responsive, and so far, she seemed to relate to us quite well. We played with the charming girl as we chatted with Melissa, trying to get as much information as we possibly could out of this encounter.

Natalie continued to be amused by our interaction until very suddenly, a switch flipped. Her tiny face transformed as though a lemon had been inserted. A cry with a level of volume unexpected for a 12 pound baby burst out of her down-turned mouth as her tongue visibly vibrated within.

"Wow, what happened?" I said, looking to Melissa for guidance.

"Oh, she's probably hungry," Melissa said as she handed me a bottle.

I placed Natalie's head in the crook of my right arm, and fed her the bottle. She immediately quieted down, eagerly sucking. Whew, that was a relief! However, ten seconds hadn't elapsed before Natalie was squirming and sour-faced once again, swatting at the bottle with a look of disgust. I pulled back the bottle.

"Oh, she's like that with feeding." Melissa said, "You have to hold her arms firmly and really force the issue to get her to stick with it."

Awkwardly, I wedged her left arm against my body and caught her flailing right arm in my right hand. Keeping a firm hold, I offered her the bottle once again. Sure enough, she relaxed and took the bottle. I was grateful to have access to a Natalie-expert, but sad that I had to consult someone else in order to do something as simple as a feeding.

After drinking her bottle, Natalie resumed squirming, and I placed her on the floor. The moment her tummy hit the blanket, she scooted herself across the room to a toy, which she grabbed and vigorously shook. I was amazed by her mobility, quite impressive for a five-month old baby! Natalie proceeded to flit from toy to toy, exploring and touching everything in her path.

Little Jack hopped about the room, and Natalie watched him, cackling with laughter. The mutual admiration between Natalie and her foster brother was unmistakable. My stomach turned at the thought of breaking up this happy little family. From my recent years of unwanted experience, I knew too well the pain and loss that I would be leaving in my wake today.

Despite the fact that the end result of our visit would inevitably inflict pain on Melissa, she was immensely gracious. The three of us actually got along well. I was so happy that Natalie had had an excellent placement for these first important months of her life. I hoped that Melissa was at least reassured that Natalie would be going to a loving family who deeply wanted her. We also made it clear that Melissa was welcome to keep in touch with us and with Natalie. We figured that some day, Natalie would want to hear stories about what she was like when she was a tiny infant. Natalie would undoubtedly want to know these people who had given her such a good start in life.

We were enjoying each others' company so much that we almost didn't notice one important detail. The social worker had not shown up! About two hours into the visit, she finally saw fit to call Melissa and explain her absence. Having left Natalie's paperwork until that very day, she was now having trouble with the computer. Apparently our licensing status was listed as Emergency Foster Care instead of Fost-Adopt. In order to complete the necessary paperwork, she needed someone from Santa Clara County to change our status on their computer system. However she was unable to get in touch with anyone in Santa Clara. She informed us that we may have to postpone Natalie's transition. The surface of my skin took a ten degree leap. How could she have left these details to the last minute? Why couldn't one thing in this train wreck of a process just go smoothly?

After all that we had been through to get to this point, I was not about to go home without Natalie. I whipped out my cell phone and called every number that I had to people who worked in Santa Clara County social services. I left messages in at least five voicemail boxes hoping that someone I reached could find a way to get into the computer and change our status.

As we waited for any word back from any social services employee from any county, Melissa's husband arrived home. Jack Sr. was a broad, burly man in a well-worn mechanic's uniform. He greeted us with a jovial smile as Jack Jr. sprung into his arms. Natalie scooted toward the gentle giant as well. Jack scooped up the grinning girl with one arm. Daddy was home.

As we spoke with Jack, I could see why Natalie smiled so much in his presence. He knew all the tricks to make her laugh, to calm her when she cried. Jack was friendly with us, but I could sense the tension inside of him as he prepared to let Natalie go.

Around 30 minutes later, Natalie's illustrious worker called back stating that Ruben, our licensing worker, had come through for us and straightened everything out. Finally, she arrived with the placement papers which we hastily signed. By this time, poor Melissa had been hosting us for over three hours! Exhausted, James and I began to pack up to leave. Jack took Natalie into his arms to say goodbye. As Natalie's mouth widened into a lop-sided smile, Jack's mouth quivered, his teeth clenched over his lower lip. Handing Natalie to James, he looked down, wiping his eyes with the sleeve of his now empty arm. Melissa remained stoic, possibly saving her tears for a later time, when house was quiet, and the reality of the loss would sink in.

We thanked them for everything, exchanged hugs, snapped a few pictures, and went on our way. As I strapped Natalie into the car seat, she stared at me with a quizzical expression. Natalie continued to stare as we drove off, no doubt wondering who the heck these people were that were taking her for a ride. I stared back at her, trying to absorb the fact that this beautiful, yet unfamiliar face, was the face of my child. The space between yesterday and today had grown our family so suddenly. It was a challenge for my mind to wrap itself around this new reality.

After a few minutes of peaceful driving, Natalie started squirming and whimpering. It didn't take her long to progress to full-on screaming. My heart raced. I was not her mommy for these first five months. I did not know how to comfort her. Melissa had mentioned that she didn't like her hair to be touched, so I stayed away from that. I offered her a bottle, which she duly rejected. James turned on some children's music in the car hoping to catch her attention. The screams continued, and the sourness of her expression steadily increased. My heart broke for her as our car moved her further and further from familiarity and comfort. Not knowing what else to do, I took her hand and just held it. After a couple more minutes of on and off crying, she settled down and drifted to sleep, her striking eyelashes curling over her dreaming eyes. I wondered where her dreams had taken her and how long it would be before her new family would join her in that world.

Jesse had been staying with James' sister while we were in Fresno. We drove straight there to pick him up and introduce him to his new sister. I wondered how he was going to react to the abrupt end of his tenure as the baby of the family. I locked my eyes onto his face as we walked in with Natalie. He calmly smiled and made his way over for a close-up view.

"Baby." he stated as I squatted on the floor with Natalie in my arms. As he approached, I feared that he would reprise his standard baby-who's-not-me-in-Mom's-arms reaction, which consisted of throwing his weight against me and frantically whining, "Up-ee, up-ee Mommy!" However this time his focus was solidly placed upon the squirmy bundle in my arms. I may as well have not been in the room. He gently touched her face and hair. The pacifier in his mouth looked out of place, as his movements made him seem suddenly like a much older child - a protective big brother. Natalie looked up at Jesse and smiled. She reached out for him too, but with much less sophistication, inadvertently swatting him in the face. I braced myself for Jesse to dissolve into tears and end the reverie of the moment, but he just carried on soaking up his baby sister as though nothing had happened. The two gazed at each other with an expression of what can only be described as recognition. The encounter had an almost eerie feel of a reunion rather than a first meeting.

As an adoptive mother, the natural tendency is to believe that blood is meaningless, that love is the sole force which bonds people together. Watching these two children made me wonder. Did they somehow have a sense of the blood that they had in common? Did they see a piece of themselves in the other, a link back to their ancestors? Or were they two people who just happened to click immediately - a random case of love at first sight? Whatever it was, the connection there could not have been more evident if glowing beams of light visibly bridged the space between their two hearts. I didn't know what forces were at work here, but I knew one thing without a shadow of a doubt. We were doing the right thing by adopting Natalie. I already could not imagine our family without her.

During her first day and evening with us, Natalie did not show any sign of panic at the sudden disappearance of her family. She happily played, intrigued by all of the new things to see. James and I interacted with her well past 9:30, long after Jesse had been tucked in for the night. I was already five months behind in getting to know her, so I felt like I wanted to drink her in all at once. Melissa had also indicated that putting Natalie to bed could be a tricky process, so I wanted her good and tired before attempting to put her down. When I could not put bedtime off any longer, I put her in pajamas and fed her a bottle. Exhausted from the long day, her eyelids drooped and sagged until even the strongest burst of willpower could not lift them off of her glazed-over eyes. I placed her in her crib, which we had set up in our bedroom, and she didn't budge even the slightest. What a relief!

I hastily got myself ready for bed so that I could grab some sleep while it was available for the taking. But before I could gingerly slither under the covers, I heard a frantic scream. To my surprise, it was not coming from the crib in my bedroom! James and I rushed to Jesse's room. We found him standing up in his crib with a horrified expression on his face. As I lifted him up, his body felt too warm against mine. He shrieked and flailed, barely able to catch his breath from one cry to the next.

"What's wrong?" We questioned him. "Does something hurt?"

But the screams were the only response that he could muster. We gave him some Tylenol, hoping that he would settle down as the fever diminished, but the intensity of his agony remained at full blast. After an hour or so of trying to calm him, we decided that we had no choice but to take him to the Emergency Room.

So at midnight, my mom rushed over to stay with Natalie (who was peacefully sleeping through all of the commotion) and James, Jesse, and I headed for the ER. Recalling horror stories from others about ER wait times, I fully expected that we would be there for the remainder of the night. However, within two hours, we were on our way to the 24-hour pharmacy with a diagnosis of a double ear infection and a prescription for antibiotics.

Natalie awakened for the first time moments before we arrived home with Jesse. His tummy filled with Motrin and antibiotics, Jesse was now relaxed and ready to sleep. I fed Natalie a bottle as James put the exhausted boy down in his crib. Natalie went back to sleep nicely, and James and I finally settled into bed to rest up for the next round. Natalie was up again at 4:00, but again went back down easily after some milk. Another two hour snooze completed the night. Welcome back, sleep deprivation!

Chapter 30
Surprise!

As Natalie settled into our home, naptime and bedtime became more similar to what Melissa had described to us. Natalie resisted sleeping with all of her might no matter how exhausted she became. She would literally smack herself in the face to try to wake herself up whenever she started to drift off. Then she would cry for long periods of time, and it was very difficult to calm her. She would refuse the bottle knowing that it would make her go to sleep. Melissa's strategy had been to put her in her swing and let her cry until she was so worn out that she would take a bottle and go to sleep. I didn't want to divert too much from what Natalie was used to, but I was not comfortable letting her cry and withholding comfort when she had so recently been ripped away from all that was familiar to her. So James and I would end up spending the nights pacing the floor, bouncing Natalie in our arms. It was the only thing that worked at all to calm her, although she would often scream through the bouncing as well.

When we weren't trying to make her sleep, Natalie was an exceedingly delightful baby. She smiled generously and played independently. She thrived on interaction, and was a highly responsive, all-around fun baby. The only thing that really made her mad was any form of sitting still. Being strapped into a car seat or a stroller was unacceptable and would elicit non-stop screaming. If we were to hold her, she would tolerate it under certain, very particular constraints. First, we had to position her facing out so that she could see the world. She required a person holding her to move in some way at all times – walking, bouncing, or swaying. This holding could only take place for a limited period of time before the urge to move and explore overtook her, and she had to be released. This was a sharp contrast to Jesse, who if he had his druthers, would still be plastered to my chest 24-7 in an infant sling. I figured Natalie's aversion to holding had to do with her generally squirmy nature and possibly with some tactile sensitivity due to the drug exposure. So I started doing daily infant massage with her, hoping to smooth out her nervous system. Natalie's mobility and squirminess made infant massage a trickier proposition than it was for Jesse. However, after a few days, she got to the point where she would enjoy it for at least a few minutes before something else caught her attention, and she scurried away.

As Jesse became more accustomed to having a baby sister, his gentle manner with her fell by the wayside, and wild excitement took its place. He loved to make her laugh, but he also loved to knock her over and poke his fingers at her eyes. We had to watch him very closely with her to ensure that she would survive infancy.

Three days after Natalie's arrival, I woke up in the morning drowsy from another difficult night. I made my way to the bathroom at the persistent urging of my bladder. Right before opening the flood gates, I stopped myself as a heart-stopping thought occurred to me. I looked at the date on my watch and counted back. It couldn't be. No, there must be some mistake. Even in the haze of sleep deprivation, I remembered back clearly the day that I ovulated. Every time I calculated it, today was 16 days from that date, two more than usual. My period was late.

Much to my bladder's protest, I clenched tightly and rushed over to the drawer to grab one of the extra pregnancy tests that I had lying around. I wrestled it out of its container and finally let my bladder have at it. The first little line popped up, closely followed by the tell-tale second line. I looked around the room making sure that there was nothing out of place to indicate that I was still dreaming. No, I was pretty sure that this was real. After eight months and multiple failed IUI attempts, in my throw- away cycle before getting started with IVF, during the intensely stressful past month, the thing that I least expected had happened. I was pregnant.

My unexpected pregnancy left James and me courting the entire spectrum of emotions with no idea which one would steal the next dance. Joy held the early lead as we marveled at our incredible little miracle. After months of tireless effort, it had finally happened naturally, the way it was supposed to happen, with no doctors anywhere in the vicinity. Scratching our heads, we wondered which night 2 ½ weeks ago had been that magical night of passion which had rescued our bank account from a $20,000 ravaging by the IVF clinic. Relief sailed atop a long, deep exhale as we pictured all of the money that wouldn't be lost, all of the needles that wouldn't be piercing my skin, and all of the doctor visits that wouldn't be taking precious time from our children. Our lives began to make sense for a change. We finally were staking our claim to a small piece of the beautiful mural of humanity that fate was lovingly painting. Perhaps there was a reason that this moment had been withheld until now. Maybe it was to ensure that we would fulfill our destiny by adopting Natalie. Now that we had these two children who were clearly meant for us, maybe this infertility curse would be lifted. As soon as my mind sashayed down that dangerous path, terror abruptly cut in with a reminder of all of the times that I had generously credited fate with finally setting things right. But each time, the results were worse than I could have imagined. The cold fact was that this pregnancy might not be any different from the others. I shuddered at the realization that I could find myself staring down the D&C machine in just a few short weeks. Further, if we failed with this pregnancy, it would be a more sharply agonizing reality to face because at that point we would have exhausted all of our options. We would have nothing left to try.

As the day to day reality started to show its face, I became more overwhelmed with the thought of facing all of these demons again alongside all of the other pressures in life. How did we expect to handle this pregnancy when we just got a new baby only three days ago! We weren't even sleeping through the night yet! Would I be spending my days and nights bouncing a screaming Natalie in one arm and a dangerously full barf-bag in the other? How would I learn all I needed to know about this precious girl with so many other thoughts swarming around my head?

I couldn't wallow in confusion for too long because there was business to take care of. Dr. Tolnai had recommended that upon a positive pregnancy test, I should get another ten days of IV antibiotics just in case there were any straggling bacteria left over. So the following Monday, I boarded a red-eye flight to JFK, grabbed a subway train to Dr. Tolnai's clinic, got the IV inserted, and returned to the airport for an afternoon flight home, missing less than one full day with Natalie. The next day, I reported to Dr. Brewer's clinic for another round of IVIG. With all of these treatments on board, I felt like maybe now we had the winning combination to make this happen. At this point, it was just another waiting game.

We continued to bond with Natalie, growing more enchanted by her every day. She continued to make an enemy of sleep, resulting in endless, intensely frustrating nights and naptimes. I desperately wanted to solidify the bond with Natalie by being present for her during the night, but at the same time, I knew that sleep deprivation would be toxic to my already precarious pregnancy. As a result, James did a large portion of the night-time feeding and pacing ritual. I even slept in a different room, trying to ignore the muffled screaming coming from down the hall. The guilt I felt over abandoning James to that excruciating struggle barely let me sleep anyway.

When I was six weeks along, I missed a call while changing Natalie's diaper. It was Mina from Dr. Brewer's clinic letting me know the results of the blood test I had taken that morning. I listened as she left a message, asking me to call the clinic. My heart rate accelerated. Why didn't she just tell me the result on the machine? Was there something wrong? It couldn't be, I reasoned as I dialed the phone. Even my shortest pregnancy so far had made it to seven weeks. I had never even seen a hint of trouble at this stage.

"Hello Julie," Mina's voice sounded hesitant. "Your hcg and progesterone levels came back this afternoon." Her next four words fired off like gunshots. "Unfortunately, they have dropped."

I knew enough about pregnancy by this point to know that hcg levels do not drop at six weeks. There is cause for alarm if they don't *double* every two to three days. I didn't have to ask Mina what this meant. Our miracle pregnancy was over. Gone before it really even started. All of the treatments I'd gone through, the thousands of dollars we had spent for them, the thousands of miles we had traveled for them had been for absolutely nothing. We didn't even make it as long as any of the previous pregnancies. After five years of singular focus, painful procedures, desperate prayers, it was all over. And we had nothing to show for it but six dead babies.

Mina suggested that I stop the progesterone supplements, and just wait for the miscarriage to happen naturally. It was too early to need a D&C. As I set the phone down, the only sound that I could hear was my pulse hammering relentlessly at my inner ear. The kids were quiet, the birds stopped singing. I don't know how much time passed as I stood there trying not to absorb what I had just heard. But the reaction had already been set in motion, and Mina's words penetrated my being like salt on a snail. I stood still, dissolving. Wasn't there some way that I could wiggle my way back in time and skip that instant when Mina's words entered my ear? Couldn't my world just rewind five minutes back to when I was safe and hopeful? Couldn't I just curl up there and live out the rest of my days?

A tug at my pant leg broke the trance. I looked down, and there was Natalie gazing up at me with a concerned look on her face. She had scooted across the room to the place where I stood. I lifted her up and held her closely. I closed my eyes as a steady stream of tears began its descent. Jesse also sensed the anguish in the air, and he came to me.

"Mommy, are you OK?" He asked.

"Yes, sweet boy." I answered as I lifted him with my free arm and received a double hug. Of course I wasn't OK, but my children's sweet display of love and concern effectively put OK back on my radar.

I called James at work. By this point, my husband and I were far from newbies when it came to receiving terrible news. Yet I had become accustomed to a particular manner of delivery. I would lie on the table, hand in hand with James as the doctor, assisted by the smarmy ultrasound machine would condemn us both to hard time in the dark, unforgiving abyss. This time was different. I would have to reach up across the border between darkness and light, and drag my unsuspecting husband back down with me. I realized that every moment that I stalled was one more moment that James could live in the blissful world of rewind that I so longed for. But that world didn't and couldn't exist. And I knew that I couldn't exist alone in my world for long. So I picked up the phone and did what had to be done. James rushed home, and we huddled together with our children, like penguins in a winter storm.

"It's over," I said, as I rested my cheek on James' shoulder. "I can't do this again."

The bleeding and cramping came within a couple of days. This time I would not have the aid of a D&C procedure to get the large chunks of pregnancy tissue out of my uterus. The pain would come suddenly and intensely, and I would buckle over, sweating. One night as I was feeding Natalie in the middle of the night, I started passing a large piece of tissue. Sitting still so as not to disturb my almost sleeping Natalie, I suppressed the urge to scream and writhe. I was struck with the irony of it all. Here I was feeding one baby as my body coldly expelled another.

I thought that it was hard to handle pregnancy with two small children, one of whom was on a sleep strike. How much more frustrating it was to carry the same load in the midst of a lost pregnancy. As Natalie screamed and fussed at night, I would hold her firmly and bounce with her, like the classes on parenting drug-exposed babies had suggested. But frequently after hours of complete ineffectiveness at calming her, the frustration would crescendo to rage. I would fantasize about holding my hand over her mouth, pressing harder until the crying just stopped. Despite my efforts to seal off the rage, every once in a while I would suddenly realize that my hold on Natalie was past the point of firm, and much more closely resembling tight. Catching myself, I would release my grip and stroke her hair, praying that she had not detected my anger. I started to understand how it happens that people commit acts of child abuse. I was teetering on the brink despite my well-adjusted childhood and supportive husband and family. With one fewer of these positive factors harnessing me to the slippery edge of that fine line, I could easily imagine stumbling over into very dangerous territory. I shamefully realized that I was no better than those people whose glassy-eyed mug shots appear on the ten o'clock news, as horrified viewers wonder how a human being could sink so low as to hurt an innocent baby. I was one small step away from being one of them. What was wrong with me? Did my maternal ineptitude span both the inside and outside of my womb?

In the days that followed, I continued to bleed as my doctors each weighed in on the meaning of this loss. Both Dr. Tolnai and the Brewer Clinic agreed that there was no apparent reason for this to happen. My NK test results had come back completely normal, and I had no symptoms of infection. I had been doing all of the immune treatments and the antibiotics they had prescribed which should have protected the baby even if infection or immune response had been present. They both agreed that the only explanation for this miscarriage was a chromosomal defect in the baby. This, they agreed, was my first pregnancy loss which truly was due to random bad luck – a bad egg or faulty fusing of the egg and sperm. Well, it's supposed to happen in one out of six pregnancies, and this was my sixth, so maybe I was due for one. Despite my battered body urging me to quit, the doctors encouraged me to give it one more try. If I went ahead with IVF, like I had been planning anyway, then I could remove the possibility of a chromosomal problem by having the embryos genetically tested prior to transferring them.

As much as James and I wanted to stop, we realized that if we didn't give it one more try, we would always wonder if we should have. And with me already 32 years old, my eggs were getting older by the second. We couldn't afford to take any breaks. So we signed on to go forward with the IVF that we had been planning. So much for the notion that our money or our hearts were safe from another round of pillaging.

Chapter 31
IVF

Before an IVF cycle can even begin, the patient must first grant her ovaries a three week vacation by taking birth control pills. A lot will be asked of said ovaries in the coming cycle. Next, she takes various medicines which prepare the uterine environment and stimulate the ovaries to work like hell to produce the maximum possible number of eggs. The doctor closely monitors the growth of the follicles, and at the optimal time, surgically removes all of the eggs from the ovaries in a procedure called the retrieval. The mature eggs are then fertilized with the father's sperm. Some will fertilize and grow. Others won't. Then, if the patient chooses, the surviving embryos can be genetically tested four days after retrieval to determine if they are chromosomally normal. This test is called pre-implantation genetic screening, or PGS. On the day following the PGS, the best of the chromosomally normal embryos are selected and transferred directly into the patient's uterus.

In order for an IVF cycle to work, everything must be planned with a great deal of precision. Each IVF patient receives a calendar, which shows the various drugs that she must ingest or inject each day of her cycle. It is a demanding schedule which requires a great deal of organization and attention to detail. On many days of my cycle, I would have up to five medications to inject at night, and upwards of ten pills to swallow over the course of the day between my IVF and immune-related meds. One might expect to find this really overwhelming, but I surprisingly found the demanding schedule to be quite comforting. Being infertile takes so much of the control out of your life. Performing the daily responsibilities of an IVF cycle actually made me feel like I had a measure of control. I was incrementally moving myself closer to the accomplishment of my goal, preparing a place inside for my baby. For me, being in cycle was a joyful time of anticipation.

My retrieval procedure took place in late June 2008. We had been tracking the growth of 21 follicles in my ovaries via ultrasound and hoping that we would get close to that many eggs from the retrieval. As it turned out, we surprisingly ended up with 32 eggs! Dr. Zoumis was astonished. Apparently, there were some additional follicles in there that were shy of the ultrasound. I could hardly blame them. I also try to hide from ultrasound machines whenever possible.

Five days later, James and I returned to Dr. Zoumis' office for the transfer. Dr. Zoumis sat us down and went over the fertilization report. Out of the 32 eggs that were retrieved, 17 had been mature. Out of those 17, 14 had successfully fertilized. The PGS testing revealed that among the 14 embryos, there were five abnormal, six completely normal, and three that Dr. Zoumis called "swing" embryos. The swing embryos each appeared to be missing one chromosome, but it was possible that they actually had one on top of another that the test did not detect. All of the six normal embryos were of extremely high quality. In fact, three of them were rated as high as an embryo can possibly be – perfect in quality, and already fully expanded blastocysts. Dr. Zoumis gushed over our embryos, saying that he only sees a result this fantastic maybe once a year.

We decided to transfer two of the best embryos, one male and one female. We would freeze the remaining normal and swing embryos. If this cycle didn't result in a pregnancy, then we would not have to start over again from scratch. Instead we could do a frozen embryo transfer. If this cycle was successful, then in a few years, we might want to try for another pregnancy using the frozen embryos. Although the eggs inside of me were constantly aging, our embryos were literally frozen in time with eggs from a 32 year old. If we were done having children before using all of the frozen embryos, we imagined that we might donate them to another couple rather than having them discarded. Every one of our children, no matter how many cells they had, were important to us.

The transfer procedure was quick and painless, except for having to keep an uncomfortably full bladder. We left the clinic with a good feeling. Two exceptionally perfect embryos were alive inside of me, burrowing their way into my uterine lining. We had given those embryos the best possible start. We had ensured that the chromosomes were normal. We had prepared my uterine environment with medications which optimally thickened the lining. We had safeguarded against immune reactions with immune treatments. We had eliminated any straggling bacteria with antibiotic treatments. We had even ventured outside of Western medicine with fertility-targeted acupuncture treatments over the course of the cycle. Nothing within our control had been left to chance. Now we just had to wait and see if chance would lighten up and cut us some slack for once.

The nice thing about a five-day transfer is that by the time the embryos are transferred, you are already two weeks, five days pregnant (since pregnancy weeks are deceptively counted from the date of the last menstrual period). So I only had to wait ten days instead of the typical two full weeks to find out the result.

I didn't like being at the mercy of the nurse who calls with the result, so I cheated and took a pregnancy test six days after the transfer. It was positive! Not just positive, but really solidly positive! The nurse called with the official blood test result four days later and informed me that my beta hcg was 442. This was almost four times higher than my beta hcg results at this stage of previous pregnancies! Looking down at my belly, I wondered how many occupants were in there. With such high numbers, I was convinced that both embryos had taken.

Over the next few weeks, my beta hcg numbers continued to soar. I became sicker as each day passed which helped me to feel secure that things were progressing. Every day at work, I would throw up at some time over the course of the day, always thanking my lucky stars that I worked at such an early hour. No one was ever in the restroom to overhear my undignified sound effects.

We had our first ultrasound at seven weeks. Dr. Truman confirmed what I had been thinking. There were two little beating hearts inside of my belly! James and I were overjoyed! If this could just work for us, we would have our boy and our girl, and we would be done with this nonsense forever. If this could just work, I thought, I could forget all of the pain and not think one more thought about fertility in my entire life.

Our second ultrasound, at 9 ½ weeks, went equally well. We sat in awe as we watched our gummy bear shaped babies squirming around in their little sacs. We had never made it to this point in pregnancy, so we had never seen our babies moving their little bodies around. They were not just blobs with flickering hearts, but actual lively beings, exploring their world.

When we reached our third ultrasound, at 11 ½ weeks, I was already starting to feel a lot less nauseous. I wasn't worried about it though because I was so near the second trimester that it actually was normal to start feeling better at this point. Dr. Truman focused on one of the twins right away. It no longer looked like a gummy bear, but like a full-fledged baby! It had a face and arms and legs, and it was moving around the sac like crazy. Dr. Truman was using a high resolution ultrasound machine that day, and James and I could have sworn that we saw some resemblance to my father in the baby. After taking several measurements, Dr. Truman moved over to Twin B. The moment I saw the sac, I knew that we would not be leaving the clinic with our hearts in working order today.

"This one is gone." Dr. Truman said flatly. "I'm sorry."

I stared at the screen not wanting to believe my eyes. Our once squiggly gummy bear was motionless, floating helplessly in its sac. Just when I was starting to think that

IVF

things might actually be OK, another baby's soul was snatched away. Why was this happening? And what did this mean for our baby who still lived?

As was the usual case, Dr. Truman didn't have any answers to our questions. She explained to us that we would just have to wait and see what happened. Twin B might just stay there and gradually shrink while Twin A grew. Or my body might try to expel Twin B which could pose a serious risk to Twin A. Even aside from how my body decided to handle the demise of Twin B, I had to wonder if whatever force killed Twin B in the first place was now headed over to Twin A to produce the same effect. Dr. Truman tried to emphasize the fact that Twin A was doing very well, and at 11 ½ weeks, was past the most typical danger zone for miscarriage. But clearly my pregnancies were not even on the same planet as *typical*. Comparisons could not be made with normal or even with abnormal pregnancies. James and I were in no-man's land and completely at the mercy of my broken-down, alien body.

The one-week wait for the next ultrasound was excruciating. We grieved for the baby we lost, and desperately feared for the baby inside. I wasn't sure if I wanted the time to pass quickly or not. This, I thought, could be my last week ever of being pregnant. Part of me wanted to stay here forever, stroking my now noticeable pregnancy bump, playing and replaying my mental picture of squirming possibility. I wanted to keep my mind safe from the image of the little person, with my father's face, staring blankly at me, floating motionless in space.

Time, however, had other ideas, and would not accommodate my desire to cling to fantasy. We found ourselves face to face with the ultrasound once again the following week. The room was silent as Dr. Truman searched for signs of life in my abdomen. She first located the grave of Twin B, lingering there and taking measurements. The baby, still hanging in space, had gotten darker in color and seemed to have reduced in size. But it appeared to be staying put next to Twin A.

"Is there a heart beat?" James asked hesitantly.

"No," Dr. Truman replied. "There's no heart beat."

With a look of shock, James slumped over, resting his face on his hand, holding my hand tightly with the other.

Wait a second. Which baby is she talking about? We are looking at the twin that was already dead right? Why isn't she looking at the healthy baby?

I had to interject at this point, "You haven't looked at Twin A yet, right?"

"That's right. This is the twin that was already gone." She responded, as James took a breath, flipping the station from utter devastation back to terrified hope.

Was Dr. Truman stalling because she was afraid to take a look at Twin A and deliver more horrendous news? Or did she just want to get the grim part of looking at the dead baby over with in the beginning? Whatever her reasons, I didn't think I could stand the wait any longer. I held on, my shallow breaths barely maintaining a hazy state of dizziness, inches from the threshold to unconsciousness. Finally, she finished her dark visit with Twin B and started making her way over to the answer that we had come for today. Twin A's sac entered the screen of the ultrasound machine. I intently focused on looking for a flickering heart, but the first thing I saw was a foot. At that point, the heart became irrelevant because the screen displayed a foot which was in the midst of a powerful, definitive kick. The rest of the body came into view, and joined the foot in playful, lively animation, announcing to the world that Baby A was unquestionably here with us.

Dr. Truman did some measurements, confirming that the Mighty Baby A was right on schedule. My heart rate slowed, and the haze around my head began to dissipate. James and I returned to the state of tempered relief which always accompanied a successful ultrasound. We had been granted a stay of execution. The immediate danger was over, though the outcome next time around was no less uncertain. But I had to admit it - 12 ½ weeks and a live baby sounded promising to me.

Chapter 32
One with the Universe

For the first time in years, the Universe and I marched together, perfectly in sync. My nausea was gone. The kids were sleeping well and becoming increasingly delightful each day as their nervous systems gradually calmed.

Week 14 brought us another successful ultrasound. Dr. Truman even got a timely little peek between the legs. She was 80-90% sure that I was carrying a little girl.

That same week brought a milestone that I had been dreaming about my entire life. I felt the baby's first definitive kick. This moment was an incomparable triumph. No matter what the future held, I would not have to live the rest of my life never having experienced that miracle.

Since we couldn't call a baby girl Isaac, and we already had our Natalie, James and I were faced with the task of coming up with another girl's name. For the first time since before we were married, we reopened the name negotiations. I suggested, and he rejected. He suggested, and I rejected. Then one day, I asked him what he thought of a name that had just popped into my mind - Ellia. I had only heard the name once before, but it had struck me that it was quite lovely, and I had tucked it away in my hit-or-miss memory bank. James liked it instantly as well. It was pretty, simple, yet quite uncommon. It could also be cutely shortened to Ellie which we both liked. When I looked the name up on a baby name website, I learned of its origin. It is a shortening of the name Elliana which means "God responded." I couldn't imagine a name more fitting. Ellia was quite literally the answer to every prayer we had uttered in the past five years.

The following week, James and I returned to Fresno with Natalie to attend the court hearing for her adoption. Unlike Jesse's adoption, Natalie's had gone through very quickly and painlessly (the Universe being on our bandwagon at this point). Natalie squirmed and wriggled as the judge echoed the words that we had heard at Jesse's hearing a little over a year ago. She was ours, and we were hers. Thank God.

My belly was sticking out considerably at this point. I had been afraid to buy maternity clothes thus far, and had just picked up a few loose-fitting items which I figured I could wear just as well in a non-pregnant state. However, it was getting to the point at which I was down to two or three outfits which I could still comfortably fit into. Luckily, my sister-in-law came through with several bags of maternity clothes which had been passed around through all of the ladies in the family, quietly skipping past me up until now.

Opening these bags of clothing, I felt like a child on Christmas. I carefully sorted through the clothes, separating the ones which would fit now from the ones I would be happily waddling around with in a few months. I even pulled out my scarcely used ironing board for the occasion, getting everything ready for wear. Skinny clothes packed away in the garage, my closet now housed my fat future which I could not wait to embrace.

At around 16 weeks, people began to notice my unmistakable bump with enough confidence to ask me when the baby was due. Each time this happened, the gleeful music in my head swelled in a glorious crescendo. I was coming out of the shadows. I was entering the world where the other women lived. I got to tell people when my baby girl would be making her appearance into the world. March 16. Five days after what would undoubtedly be my best birthday ever.

My friends whom I met in Nogales were also reaping the rewards of the miraculous fertility treatments. Abby had given birth to a baby boy. Chloe and Lorraine each had twin boys. Sendy and had a baby girl. Most of these babies were already over a year old. Debby, the only one in the group who had also gone to Dr. Tolnai, had just given birth to a healthy baby girl. Out of all of the couples I kept in contact with from the Nogales trip, Roma, who had unfortunately miscarried her post-Nogales pregnancy, was the only one who was still unsuccessful. Maya, the woman I had met in Dr. Brewer's office that first day, had also had a textbook pregnancy resulting in a beautiful little girl. That's a pretty amazing record, considering that we were all lost causes to conventional medicine a little over two years ago. As week 17 brought another successful ultrasound, I looked forward to announcing our happy news on the Immunology boards and adding to the success stats of Dr. Brewer and Dr. Tolnai.

Chapter 33
Cramped

When I was 18 weeks along, James and I went in for our level two ultrasound. This was the first ultrasound that I actually wasn't dreading. We had had a successful ultrasound only one week prior, and I was feeling Ellie squirming several times a day, so I knew we would be seeing her alive. Plus, this scan would be done with better equipment, so we could get a nice look at Ellie, and hopefully reconfirm that she was actually a she. James and I were even brave enough to pay the extra $20 to get a souvenir DVD of the ultrasound.

A gust of cold air entered the exam room as the stony-faced technician entered. She didn't utter a word as she applied clear jelly to my round belly and opened the window to Ellie's world. A strongly beating heart appeared on the screen. Now we just had to make sure that all of her organs were in the right places and properly sized. Much to my disappointment, despite the larger, fancier machine, the images were not clearer than last week's. In fact, it seemed considerably harder to make things out. Maybe it was because Ellie was so much bigger now. It was harder to get a good view of her because she filled so much of the space at this point. The curved line of her spine made her look like she was tightly curled up in there. I shrugged. That must be why they call it "fetal position."

"That is the brain." The technician's monotonic voice broke the silence.

"I'm glad that's in the right place," I said, smiling at James.

The technician didn't crack a smile. I wondered if she practiced a vacant expression in front of a mirror each morning. She returned to silence. I knew that technicians were not supposed to comment on anything, leaving the analysis of the images to the doctor. Still, this woman did a better robot than R2D2.

"These are the kidneys." The Sonogra-bot managed another utterance.

I couldn't resist asking. "Does everything look normal so far?"

"The kidneys look normal."

OK, I actually asked about "everything", not just the kidneys.

The technician must have been trained not to make blanket statements. Something in her tone made me feel very uneasy. I decided not to ask any more questions.

She continued making measurements and typing on the screen. I watched as measurements flashed onto the screen. Everything was coming up somewhere between 17 weeks, 5 days and 18 weeks, 2 days. I didn't have to ask her to know that Ellie's growth was right on track.

Lifting the wand, the technician placed a towel over my belly. "Stay here in case the doctor wants to look some more."

Wait, she had forgotten something important! I stopped her, "Were you able to tell if it was a boy or a girl?"

"Well, I didn't get a good view," she responded, reluctantly placing the wand back on my belly. "See, here are the legs." She manipulated the wand for a second, feigning an effort to zero in on the area, then quickly removed the wand saying, "I really can't tell." She hastily left the room.

"Well the measurements all looked good." I said to James, holding his hand tightly, "Ellie must have grown a lot. She's starting to look cramped in there."

"Yeah," James responded, "She seems a lot bigger than last week."

James and I waited quietly and tensely for the doctor. The large room was dark and cold. I tried to convince myself that it was just the technician's strange vibe that had thrown things off, but I felt very unsettled, and I could tell that James did too. *Just wait for the doctor.* It seemed like waiting was all we ever did.

The door slammed into the wall as Dr. Fisher burst into the room.

"Have you had any cramping or bleeding?" He asked without even a hello.

"No," I responded.

"Why did Dr. Truman send you here for an ultrasound?" He asked. "What symptoms were you having?"

"This was just our 18 week ultrasound." I said.

"So everything was normal up until now?" He snarled incredulously.

"Well, we lost a twin early on, but everything was normal after that. Our last ultrasound was a week ago, and everything was normal." I responded.

"Well, I don't know about last week, but this is *not* normal."

The technician peeked back into the room. "Dr. Truman is on the line." She said.

My frenzied gaze darted back and forth between the technician and the doctor. The walls whirled around my head.

This can't be happening. Not after everything we've been through. There must be some mistake.

"Look at this," Dr. Fisher said with a look of disgust as he ripped off the towel and grabbed the wand. "There is hardly any fluid. The baby can barely move in there. This darker portion here is blood. I don't know if this is because of the blood thinners you've been taking, but if I were you, I would stop taking them. The baby still looks normal at this point, but it won't be for long."

"Is there anything we can do?" I asked, "Like bed rest or drinking lots of water?" I had heard of cases of people who have had a tear in the sac and leaked out amniotic fluid. They would go on bed rest and drink something like 3 gallons of water a day, and the fluid would be partially replaced until the baby was far enough along to be born.

"Well, you can try bed rest if you want." Dr. Fisher gruffly replied, "But in my experience, these problems very rarely can be corrected. And if you drink additional water, you'll just pee it out anyway."

Although, Dr. Fisher intended to be discouraging, one of his statements inadvertently gave me hope.

My tightening throat barely let my words out, "So you've seen cases like this where things have turned around?"

"Listen," he replied, taking no pains to hide his condescension, "The baby may seem normal right now, but it is the baby which produces the amniotic fluid. When that is drastically reduced, that means that there is something that has gone seriously wrong with the baby. All we can really do is watch and see what happens, but with such an abnormal placenta, I expect that things will get much worse, and quickly. You can make an appointment to come back for another ultrasound in one week."

And with that, the technician shoved into my hand the DVD we had bought, and the two left the room.

If this sensitivity-vacuum thought I would ever voluntarily come see him and his robot friend again, he had to be crazier than he was mean! It was bad enough to hear the worst news of one's life without having it delivered via steel-toed boot kicks to the head. As we unsteadily walked out of the clinic from hell, the footsteps of six other similar walks echoed across the icy walls.

James left me sitting by the front door as he walked out to bring the car. I immediately took out my cell phone to seek help from doctors who actually knew what they were doing. I first called Dr. Brewer's clinic and left a message. Next, I called Dr. Tolnai. Although it was not uncommon for Dr. Tolnai to personally answer calls to his office, his nurse picked up this time. After hearing my predicament, she routed the call directly to Dr. Tolnai. I described to him what had happened, and he recommended that I take bed rest and get IV antibiotics immediately. He assured me that cases like this can turn around and that it was not over yet. I knew that I would not be able to get a local doctor to prescribe IV antibiotics, and I obviously couldn't fly to New York. Dr. Tolnai offered to speak directly to Dr. Truman. I gave him her phone number and hoped that he could convince her.

As our minds continued on the sharp detour to darkness, the car managed somehow to deliver us safely home. James helped me into bed. As my head hit the pillow, I looked around the room. This place would be my prison, maybe for the next several months. Down in my belly, Ellie sat in her own prison. My worthless body caved in over the both of us as we crouched together.

I could hear James with the children in the next room. My mom, who had been watching them when we went for the ultrasound, was hearing a recounting of the day's horrors. My thoughts turned to my children. How were we going to take care of them with me out of commission? I knew that our extended family would rally around us, but the kids needed their parents. Natalie had just joined our family. What had I gotten us into?

Not long after I got home, Dr. Truman called. She had spoken to Dr. Tolnai, and as I fully expected, he had been unable to convince her to prescribe IV antibiotics. I asked her to explain what had happened over the past week.

"Well, it is unclear what actually happened," Dr. Truman responded, "There seems to be some bleeding from the placenta, but it is hard to tell what is going on. Dr. Fisher is calling it a placental abruption."

"Have you ever seen a case like this before?" I asked her.

"Not at this stage in pregnancy."

"I want to get a second opinion," I said to Dr. Truman. "I'd like to see a perinatologist at Stanford."

"Yes, I think it is a good idea to get a second opinion." Dr. Truman replied. "I will make a referral for you." Dr. Truman paused. "I'm so sorry this is happening. I wish there was something I could do."

I thanked her and hung up the phone, returning to the isolation of my bed. Besides her sympathy, Dr. Truman had given me one valuable thing. She had put a name to what was happening – placental abruption. I logged onto my laptop and started researching the condition. I found that placental abruption is a separation of the placenta from the uterine wall which causes bleeding that can be highly dangerous to both mother and child. It typically happens in the third trimester, and the treatment is to deliver the baby immediately. This can be very dangerous because as the baby is being delivered, the placenta can separate more, causing severe hemorrhaging, which can lead to organ failure and death. C-sections can also be dangerous, as the surgery causes additional blood loss. Bleeding of that extent can cause the blood to lose its ability to clot even when transfusions are given.

    I was only 18 weeks along, still six long weeks from Ellie being viable to deliver. And if my defective placenta was starving her bit by bit, there was little hope of her surviving that long. I began to see the inescapable path that I would be forced to walk in the near future. I was going to deliver a dead baby and perhaps die myself in the process. I thought about what that would be like – the painful contractions, the pushing, the moment when Ellie would be born, and her cries would not be heard. Would I hold her after she came out? What would she look like? Would there be a moment when her body still held the warmth of my body when it would seem like she was alive? I promised myself that even if I was bleeding to death, I would hold her and look deeply into her face. I would memorize every contour of her face and hope that time would never fade that image. I would tell her how much I loved her, and how sorry I was that I could not protect her.

    All I could do was sob into my pillow. I wanted to leap out of bed and throw things. I wanted to leap into the sky and tell God what I thought of his brilliant plan. Ellia was quite literally *God's response*, just as her name depicted. His Almighty Response to five years of nonstop praying – the drawn out death of my beautiful baby girl and perhaps the orphaning of my live children. I wanted nothing to do with this God.

    The next morning, I finally got through at the Brewer Clinic. I explained to the nurse what had happened, and as a welcome change of pace, she responded with fierce reassurance.

"Do not lose hope. We have had so many patients who have been unnecessarily distressed by Dr. Fisher. He is actually notorious around here. Many times, he has urged patients to terminate their pregnancies, and they have gone on to deliver full-term, healthy babies. Don't listen to what he says. What we typically do in these situations is three days in a row of IVIG. A lot of times that turns things right around. Just keep resting and drinking tons of water, and we can fit you in today for an IVIG treatment."

I valued the Brewer clinic's opinion over anyone else's, so if they believed that hope was not forever lost, then I was ready to lead the search party. I reported for IVIG several hours later. The attentive staff ushered me in, sympathetic, but full of fight. They relayed more horror stories that had been authored by dear Dr. Fisher. One nurse said, "When your baby is born, you should march her straight in to Dr. Fisher to show him how wrong he was." I pictured Ellie and me beating the odds and proving him wrong. As the IV infused my veins with medicine, the staff infused my spirit with resolve. I needed to stay strong and picture the best possible outcome. Ellie needed my body to be calm and working at full capacity. As long as she was kicking inside of me, this was not over.

My appointment at Stanford was the following Monday. Upon arriving, I found that the perinatologist on staff that day was Dr. Lionel. I flashed back remembering our visit with her years ago after our second loss. Five pregnancies later, here we were again, still failing. As the technician performed the ultrasound, I held up a mirror so that I could see the screen. I wondered if it was just wishful thinking, but Ellie seemed to have considerably more space than she did four days ago. Maybe she was just more relaxed out of the vicinity of Dr. Fisher. When the ultrasound was complete, Dr. Lionel entered the room, and with hushed voices, she and the technician conferenced over the images on the opposite side of the room. As I waited for their deliberation, I locked my eyes on the poster on the ceiling above the ultrasound. The peaceful image of a brilliant, blue sky filled with billowing clouds reminded me of heaven. I wondered if that was where my babies go when they leave me. Would I see them there again some day?

Finally, Dr. Lionel approached us, grasping the wand and taking a look for herself. "Well, the good news is that at this point, the baby looks fine. Every measurement, except for the femur length is right on target. The measurement which we look at to evaluate placental function is typically the abdominal circumference, which is totally fine." Dr. Lionel's pause announced the abrupt departure from good news, "However, I'm not sure what is going on in this area here." She pointed at an area at the base of the gestational sac. "The placenta is supposed to be up here, but it appears to be incredibly enlarged, extending all the way to the cervix. At this point, it is hard to tell whether this area is truly part of the placenta or if it is a hematoma. Currently, there is blood flow to the area, which would indicate that it is placental tissue. A large placenta combined with a shorter femur length can be an indication of several genetic disorders."

"But this was an IVF pregnancy," I interjected, "The embryos were all genetically tested."

"Yes," Dr. Lionel responded, "Which would make a genetic problem less likely, but still possible, since PGS is not 100% accurate. We will know more in a week or so. If this area is a hematoma, then we will start to see more of a demarcation between placental tissue and blood clot. Then we will have a better idea of what is happening."

"What about the amniotic fluid?" I asked, "Dr. Fisher said that I had barely any amniotic fluid."

"I did see that in his report," Dr. Lionel responded. "Looking at the images today, though, I am not too concerned about it. The fluid shows up on the ultrasound as the darker areas." She manipulated the wand, "You can see this pocket here is 4.7 cm, which is pretty good. At worst, I would characterize the fluid as low normal. I'm not sure what Dr. Fisher saw the other day, but what I am seeing today is dramatically different from what he described. I suppose it is possible that the IVIG treatment could account for this improvement."

Dr. Lionel recommended continuing bed rest, IVIG, and fluids. We scheduled a follow-up in a week. As James pushed my wheelchair out the door of the clinic, the smell of doom in the air was slightly less overpowering than it had been when we entered. Hope, like a dangerous drug, tantalized us, daring us to plunge it into our fiending veins.

I followed the doctor's orders to the letter. My feet only made contact with the floor on Nature's marching orders (which were issued with greater-than-average frequency due to my endless chugging of the water bottle). Family rallied around us. My sister-in-law and mother-in-law prepared my favorite foods. My mother's sister flew in from New York to stay with us and take on the Natalie night duty. She, my mom, my grandmother, and James all worked round the clock to care for the kids and keep the household running. It was excruciating for me to relinquish my duties to others. Hearing my children cry and not being able to run to them was the worst form of torture. All I ever wanted to be was a mother, and the harder I tried to make it happen, the less of a mother I became.

As I watched my work going on around me, I did come to an oddly validating revelation. I was not easily replaced. It took an extensive team of people conscientiously working to accomplish my daily tasks – it was exhausting just witnessing it! With my weaknesses constantly paraded out for all to see, at least I had this one small consolation.

James bought me books to help pass the time, and I attempted to stay in the world of the books, outside of my mind. In order to keep my body as calm as possible, I could not entertain any thinking about my situation, good or bad. Even a split-second reflection on my gratitude toward my family would release an unstoppable tidal wave of emotion. I avoided engaging in conversation to the point of rudeness. I hoped that everyone would understand - Ellie was relying on me to keep her safe.

As days went on, I felt increasingly dingy. My skin itched and my body ached for movement. One evening, James, sensing my discomfort, arrived at my bedside, arms filled with bathing supplies. He placed plastic under my head and let my hair fall over the edge of the couch. Tenderly, he poured warm water over my hair, letting it fall into an empty basin beneath. As he massaged the shampoo into my hair, my body completely relaxed for the first time in recent memory. I could swear that I felt each hair follicle releasing a sigh of relief, one by one, as the perfectly warmed water gently massaged away the stagnation. Next James scrubbed my face, arms, and legs with a hot washcloth. Every ache and itch dissolved into the steaming vapor. I escaped for a short time to a place where nobody dies, and only love exists.

I smiled at my husband, "You're getting a sneak preview of what it will be like when I'm old." I was 1 ½ years older than James, and we had often joked about how I had robbed the cradle, and he would one day be burdened with caring for an elderly wife. If old age did leave me incapacitated someday, there was no doubt that I would be in the best of hands.

Chapter 34
Drained

The days passed excruciatingly slowly as I served my sentence. Every air molecule in the house pressed pleadingly against the walls and windows, seeking release from the corked-up tension. Book to book, couch to bathroom, consciousness muzzled, I existed.

James stayed strong around me, but I could see the strain forming a separate gravitational field around him. His shoulders and face slumped toward the floor. His goofy charm had departed to the same shadowy place where my manners had gone. Not wanting to leave my side, he could only escape for short intervals, running a quick errand or taking an occasional walk. During one of those rare occasions, shortly after he had taken a grouchy Jesse out for a nighttime stroll, I stood at the behest of my bladder and started making my way to the restroom. A couple of steps in, a sudden flash flood burst out of my body. I clenched my legs together, trying to hold back whatever it was, but the force of the fluid was too great. Like a knocked-over fire hydrant, nothing could interfere with the will of the flow. My mind sputtered, trying to get some sort of grasp on what was happening to me. Had my water broken? What the hell else could go wrong? I sprinted to the bathroom, ripping off my soaking wet pants. To my surprise, I was not bathing in amniotic fluid. I stared in horror at the river of blood that was collecting on the floor beneath my shaky feet. The shocking scene looked as though an axe murderer had paid a visit. I called for my aunt. She was putting Natalie to bed a couple of rooms down. She didn't hear me. I shouted louder. Still no response. Realizing that I needed to make contact with someone who could help me, and fast, I wrapped a towel between my legs and grabbed the nearest phone, dialing James' cell. No answer. The blood faucet still running at full force, I dashed for my cell phone which held the number for the on-call obstetrician. Recognizing that I needed to get my body near the floor before it forced me there, I headed for the kitchen, hoping to spare the carpet from becoming a part of the crime scene. On the floor, the blood flow no longer had gravity as an accomplice, and to my relief, it slowed considerably.

As I was leaving an urgent message for the doctor, my aunt finally surfaced from Natalie's room. She gasped as she realized what was happening.

All I could say was, "I need James." I knew full well that she couldn't just leave me alone with Natalie and go hunt for him, but he was the only person that I wanted with me. He was the only person who could handle this and whom I could handle seeing. At that moment, as though he had psychically heard my plea, James appeared at the front door. I tried to stay as calm as possible so as not to alarm Jesse.

"Sweetie, I'm bleeding a lot." I said. "We need to go to the hospital."

James, always clear-thinking during emergencies, sprung into action. He settled Jesse on the couch. Grabbing a maxi-pad and fresh clothing for me, he helped me get dressed and then gently carried me out to the car. We reclined the passenger seat, and I placed my feet up on the dashboard.

A couple minutes into the drive, the on-call obstetrician returned my call. He instructed us to come straight to Labor and Delivery rather than the ER. The words *labor* and *delivery* sent a fresh wave of terror through my body. Was I going to deliver my baby tonight? If she was still alive, there was no way for her to survive. I was only 19 weeks pregnant. We descended the ramp to highway 237. As if things couldn't get any worse, I started to notice the car slowing down. The next thing I knew, we had come to an ominous halt. I lifted my head and peered out the window. There were cars as far as the eye could see, and not a single one of them was moving. Was I going to deliver Ellie in the car and bleed to death in the traffic?

"What are we going to do?" I shrieked as I frantically groped for a solution to this problem. We could call 911, but how could an ambulance even get to us? Before I could come up with an alternate idea, I felt the car move once again. James had pushed the emergency lights on, swerved to the left, and sped onto the shoulder of the road. The ride was bumpy and of course highly illegal, but we were moving, and that was all that mattered. If a police officer stopped us, then all the better – our situation would have probably merited a complimentary escort.

My heroic husband delivered us to the hospital, car and occupants unscathed. He parked the car and dashed in to fetch a wheelchair. I was hesitant to sit upright and inevitably feel more blood gush out, but it was our only way in.

James wheeled me to the nurses' station at Labor and Delivery. Of course, consistent with the sadistic playbook of my life, we couldn't avoid passing by the baby nursery on the way. I averted my eyes, but my ears couldn't escape the taunting newborn noises. I seethed at the repulsive stench of bliss that hung in the air. People holding flowers and balloons craned their necks to see the new little arrivals. How out of place was I with my pathetically small belly and distant, ghostly stare? What gave every other jerk the right to my happy ending?

In the distance, we finally caught sight of the nurses' station. A couple of nurses and a doctor stood at the station, and appeared to be watching for us. As we approached, I focused in on the doctor. I took a prolonged blink, willing my eyes to see something different when my eyes reopened. But no such luck. Standing before me was none other than Dr. Gravel, the doctor/bulldozer who had referred to my first dead baby as a freak of nature, not even up to heaven's standards.

I shrugged. It may as well be him. What difference would it make anyway? The most sensitive, empathetic doctor in the world probably couldn't put a positive spin on this situation.

I was quickly ushered into a room, and placed into a bed. As we brought Dr. Gravel up to speed on the issues of the pregnancy, he performed a pelvic exam. My cervix was closed, so at least labor was not imminent. He said that he couldn't be sure if the sac was leaking because there was so much blood.

Next came the ultrasound. I stared at the screen, lacking the energy to plead with it to show us a beating heart. My hope of seeing anything but doom was gone. As the screen came to life, there was Ellie. My beautiful little girl was peacefully floating, wiggling her limbs, calmly doing her baby thing. She seemed completely oblivious to all of the chaos around her. I was relieved that she was still with us, but terrified of the horrors she might be forced to endure in the near future as her world was clearly unraveling around her.

"The baby seems to be doing fine for now," Dr. Gravel said. "I don't know what is causing the bleeding, but the baby is not in distress, and you are not in labor. That's a good sign. We'll admit you to the hospital and get a large-bore IV in you in case you need a transfusion. As soon as we can get an appointment, we'll have you go up to the Prenatal Diagnostic center. They have a much higher quality ultrasound machine. Maybe then we'll have a better idea of what is going on."

The nurse got me set up with an IV. She placed plastic sleeves around my legs, which constantly inflated and deflated. The incessant squeezing and unsqueezing of my legs was supposed to prevent blood clots from forming due to inactivity. Of course, as soon as I was all hooked up, I realized that I needed to use the bathroom.

"Well, we don't want you getting up and walking around." The nurse responded. "I'll bring you a bedside commode."

My dignity made a grand and stately exit as I let the nurse unplug all of my gadgets and help me to my potty chair. Each visit with the vertical started me leaking down below and bracing myself for another onslaught of the faucet. As I sat on the commode, the nurse stood in front of me holding a toilet paper roll. Ordinarily, I can be a bit timid when it comes to standing up for my personal rights, but this was where I drew the line.

"I'll call you when I'm done." I said assertively, motioning toward the nurse button.

"Oh, of course," the nurse replied, handing me the toilet paper roll and making a quick exit.

Much to my chagrin, the stress of the day had taken its toll on my digestive system, and the night brought frequent encounters with the commode and the nursing staff. The nurses never missed an opportunity to comment on what I had left for them to clean up.

"Oh, your stools are quite loose," was the common observation, followed with, "I'll have to mention that to the doctor." *Perfect, you do that. While you're at it, maybe announce it over the P.A. system, just so that everyone's aware.*

The ultimate in mortification came when several hours into the night, one of the nurses actually tripped and spilled the contents of the commode all over the floor. The custodian was no doubt combing through the want-ads after that nasty clean-up job.

I don't believe that I slept more than a few minutes at a time that entire night. My bed, which was meant for labor rather than rest, would have drawn bitter complaints from Fred Flintstone. Every part of me that made contact with the bed was either throbbing, numb, or tingling. Nurses came and went every few hours and listened to the baby's heartbeat on the Doppler. Even if I had been sleeping, it wouldn't have lasted long with all of the interruption.

Around 3:00 am, I must have dosed for a bit because I was startled awake by loud and desperate screaming. I lifted my head and looked around, but couldn't see the source of the commotion. As the screams continued, I realized that they were coming from the room next door. Muffled voices communicated urgency. The screaming started intensifying and coming in shorter intervals. It didn't take a genius to figure out what was going on. Someone was giving birth on the other side of my wall. I marveled once again at the universe's never-ending supply of wound-rubbing salt. Wrapping the rock which doubled as a pillow around my head, I tried not to listen. But it was pointless. I could hear everything – the uninhibited shrieks of the woman, the supportive encouragement of the medical staff, and finally, the vigorous entrance of the newest little voice-box on the planet. This was the story of my life. Peering in windows at other people's children. A solid, but not soundproof wall separating me from the experience that I had longed for my entire life. Was this as close as I would ever get?

The next morning, the nurse informed me that I would be moving from Labor and Delivery to the Maternity ward. Immediately, my mind flashed straight to a stomach-turning picture of smugly smiling ladies wheeling about with their cuddly new bundles, eager relatives crowding around. I would take waking to the screams of labor pains over that bliss force-feed any day. I protested to the nurse to let me stay, but when she explained that the Maternity ward came with a comfortable bed, I piped down immediately. I couldn't take any more hard time in the labor bed.

So James and the nurse wheeled me over to Maternity. As promised, the bed was quite comfortable, and I finally was able to sleep. Every once in a while, a short clip of Brahms' "Lullaby and Goodnight" would play over the intercom system. I soon caught on that they played the tune each time a baby was born back in my old neighborhood.

My mom brought Jesse and Natalie to visit me around midday. Their eyes darted anxiously as they entered the room. My mom placed Natalie on the bed next to me.

"Hi Mommy," she said as she gave me a kiss. I hugged her tightly, filling my nostrils with her sweet scent. Jesse climbed up as well and curled up next to me.

"Mommy, you have owie?" he asked, pointing to the tape on my hand which held the IV in place.

"No," I responded lightly. "That tape just holds this tube that is giving me some medicine."

My answer seemed to satisfy him, but he was still intent on rubbing his fingers across the strange tape. "You coming home Mommy?" he asked.

"Yes, the doctor said I can come home really soon." I prayed that I was telling him the truth.

The kids hadn't been with me long before Natalie started squirming. My mom lifted her up. "Eat, eat," she whined. You would never guess how much Natalie ate by looking at her. She was so thin that she had actually been diagnosed "Failure to Thrive." But thrive was a word which perfectly captured her. She never stopped moving, exploring, smiling, or talking. At only 13 months, her vocabulary was well over 100 words, and she used those words every chance she got.

"They're probably getting hungry." My mom said as she started to gather up their things. Jesse snuggled in tighter. I didn't want to let go either. The doctor entered the room, which hastened their exit. As I watched the backs of their beautiful heads moving further away from me, all I wanted was to follow them out – to go home and be their mom like I was supposed to be. If I had thought that something like this would happen, I would never have tried for another pregnancy. Why couldn't I have just let well enough alone?

Despite the torment of the incessant lullabies, my stay in the Maternity ward was relatively peaceful. I slept much better, which helped to pass the time until the ultrasound appointment finally came. With this scan, the picture inside became a bit clearer. As suspected, the placenta was not enlarged, but there was a massive hematoma which finally distinguished itself from the placenta. The baby was still doing fine. However, the doctor informed me that a hematoma of that size was intrinsically unstable and could cause labor to occur at any time. The suggestion was to continue bed rest and return for another scan in a week.

I stayed in the hospital for one more night until the bleeding had wound down to an occasional trickle. At that point, I was finally allowed to return home. I had been so singularly focused on getting out of the hospital and returning to my children, that I hadn't really given any thought to what it would be like to be home. In many ways, it was actually more stressful than being in the hospital. My kids were understandably grumpy having their mom return after many days, still totally out of commission. They were in good, loving hands, but every person caring for them was stressed to within millimeters of the breaking point. Outrageous would be too kind a term to describe Jesse and Natalie's behavior at that time. Screaming had become the new soundtrack in our home.

In addition, I found myself plagued with new worries. Being so far from the hospital, I lived in constant fear of having another bleeding episode. Every time I moved, I braced myself. To make it worse, I was still spotting and occasionally passing large clots. The doctor assured me that it was to be expected that chunks of the hematoma would be expelled from time to time. It was actually a good thing, since coming out little by little was a way to safely decrease the size of the enormous clot. But it was quite disconcerting to feel the painful cramping and not know if I was passing a clot or going into labor. I was told to come back to the hospital if the cramping were to come and go in regular intervals. It was hard to measure each interval as my uterus clamped and unclamped, working on the clots. But each time I finally passed a clot, the pain would stop. So retroactively, I could confirm that I was not in labor.

One week passed, and I returned for my follow-up ultrasound. Having expelled so many clots over the week, I was hopeful that we would see the hematoma drastically reduced in size. No such luck. It was larger. Dr. Al-Fayadh put down the wand and turned to face me.

"Julie, there is something drastically wrong with the placenta. You have had significant bleeding. The further you go with this, the more risk there is to you. You may want to seriously consider terminating this pregnancy."

What was this guy smoking? Had he actually read my chart? After five years and six miscarriages, here I was with a pregnancy that was four weeks from becoming viable. My baby girl was counting on me, and there was no chance that I was going to give up on her now.

"We are not going to terminate this pregnancy." I responded firmly, hoping to close that topic once and for all.

"You have some time to decide." The doctor continued, unwilling to leave well enough alone. "But once you hit 24 weeks, termination will no longer be an option. This pregnancy is becoming a seriously high risk to your health."

Why was he going on about risks to me? I didn't care what happened to me as long as I could bring Ellie into the world. I would do whatever it took. I reiterated to Dr. Al-Fayadh that there was no chance that I was going to terminate. Finally he let it drop.

James and I sat silently on the drive home from the ultrasound. We were entering new and ever more dangerous territory. It should have been obvious, but until Dr. Al-Fayadh forced it kicking and screaming into the light, I hadn't given any thought to the serious threat to my own health. I had been so focused on Ellie's survival that my own survival had never even entered my inner discussion. This was all just too much to process. But I knew for sure I wasn't going to give up, so that was that. Thinking about this further was simply not an option. What I needed to do was to get back to my couch and my books and put my weary brain back on hiatus.

Today, however, my books were not going to save me. Today was Halloween. This was my Jesse's absolute favorite holiday of all time. To him, Disneyland paled by comparison with a visit to the Halloween Superstore. Only a few weeks ago, I had been taking the kids for daily walks to see what new spooky decorations had appeared in the neighbors' yards. Tonight was the pinnacle of a year's worth of built up excitement. And I was going to miss the entire thing.

I labored to keep a firm grip on my tears as the kids got dressed up and took pictures. This year Jesse was big enough to wear the family monkey costume which my grandfather had sewn for my mother when she was four years old. Like all things my grandfather had made, the costume had held up tremendously well over time. It had survived previous wearings by my older brother, my younger cousin, and Marsha. Now it was Jesse's turn to carry on the tradition. The costume perfectly fit both the body and the personality of my goofy boy. Natalie bounced about the room in her Dalmatian costume. Her striking dark hair and eyes, along with her ear-to-ear grin made her a puppy that Cruella herself would find impossible to resist. Children did not come any cuter than these two. The rip in my heart lengthened with their every smile. I couldn't imagine any form of existence that didn't include those smiles.

When the front door shut behind them, I quickly picked up my book. But the tears were already hard at work blurring my escape route. I sobbed the entire time the kids were gone and much of the night that followed. There was no thought in my mind. Just emotion in its rawest form, clawing its way out.

Chapter 35
The Descent

It was the next day that I started hemorrhaging again. The faucet started spewing just as suddenly as it had the last time. James was out on an errand. My mom and the kids were the only ones with me. Dr. Gravel had advised me to call an ambulance upon another bleeding episode so that the paramedics could insert an IV for a blood transfusion in case I needed one upon arrival at the hospital. I was not thrilled at the thought of calling an ambulance, but with James gone as well, I figured we didn't have much choice. No more than a minute had passed after the 911 call when we heard the approaching sirens – apparently I lived in the right place to have an emergency. As concerned neighbors gawked from their yards, the paramedics paraded me out in all my glory. And I thought that I had no remaining dignity to lose!

Back in Labor and Delivery again, I experienced a replay of my recent hospital experience – pelvic exam, blood test, IV, ultrasound, leg squeezers, befuddled doctor. Ellie was still looking just as good. The bleeding, although it was already slowing down, was just as ominous. James had arrived at the hospital shortly after I did. We would obviously be spending another night there.

As I settled in for another all-nighter with the rock-solid labor bed, I started to realize that some measures regarding my care were up to the discretion of the particular doctor or nurse that happened to be on duty when I came in. For some reason, this particular set of hospital staff wasn't keen on the idea of me using a bedside commode for my restroom needs. The only option set before me this time was to use a bed pan. I put it off as long as possible, but eventually, I had no choice but to surrender to biological need. It would serve the inventor of the bed pan right if he were cursed to spend eternity bedridden, with nothing but his lofty invention and an endless supply of cashews and prune juice. From its icy cold metal to its astonishing ability to resist forming to any contour of the body, the bed pan could not have been designed to be any more shockingly uncomfortable. Furthermore, all muscles involved in filling the bed pan had long been programmed to keep a firm hold while the body is in a horizontal position. After 20 or so minutes of cajoling, my stubborn muscles finally relented. I dismounted, completely grossed out, hoping with all my might that the nurse would grant me one small favor and manage not to spill the contents this time.

To make matters worse, this particular nursing staff wanted me to wear a monitor around my abdomen which tracked the baby's heart rate and watched for signs of uterine contractions. The monitor was tight and uncomfortable around my belly which by this point felt heavy and achy all the time. Shortly after setting up the monitor, the nurse returned to my room with the cheery news that I was having mini-contractions. She gave me a drug called nifedipine which was supposed to settle my uterus down. My belly did feel a bit more relaxed after taking the pill. Throughout the night, I listened to the monitor as it scratched away on a strip chart next to my bed. Every time I heard its agitated scribbling, I realized that my uterus was probably acting up again. I felt as though my baby were being silently stalked by my own predator body. My heart raced helplessly as pre-term labor crouched in the nearby bushes, ready to pounce. It wasn't long before I had worked myself into a complete frenzy. The aching in my abdomen swelled to intense cramping. I buckled over in pain and reached for the nurses' button. The nurse came in and gave me another pill. The cramping soon subsided, but the rest of my body wasn't doing so well. I started feeling overwhelmed by a desperate desire to extricate myself from my own skin. I felt hot and weird all over, and my head started to throb. The nurse informed me that I was having a reaction to the nifedipine. My blood pressure had dropped suddenly. I thrashed about the bed searching for a position that would stop the stampede of creepy crawlies. The effects of the pill finally wore off after an hour or two. Thankfully, I didn't progress into labor, but after my reaction to nifedipine, I had no recourse if labor were to threaten again.

I made a decision at that point that the fetal monitor was simply not an option. Every time the nurse dutifully came in to tighten it, I waited for her to leave the room, and then I loosened it. I knew that there was nothing that could be done at this point if I went into labor or if Ellie's heart stopped beating, so why torture myself with the monitor?

With the frantic strip chart action out of my head, I was finally able to get some sleep. Somehow, the night gave way to morning. The doctor on duty that morning was Dr. Jackman, the OBGYN that I had seen for my very first pregnancy. We had come full circle.

Dr. Jackman sent me upstairs to the Stanford Diagnostic Center for another scan. I was greeted by Dr. Travers, yet another perinatologist who had never seen me before. As he adjusted the wand on my tender belly, he pointed to the ultrasound screen.

"This hematoma is really in an odd location. Usually they form on the back of the placenta. This one is actually inside the gestational sac. Since you have no tear in the sac, the hematoma could not be the source of your bleeding."

No wonder the chunks of clot that I was passing did not reduce the size of the hematoma! It was coming from somewhere else. This was an interesting revelation, but not helpful in the least. Now I was bleeding from not only one but two places, both internally and externally. Dr. Travers said that all we could do is continue on as we had been doing – waiting and hoping for the bleeding to stop at least long enough for Ellie to become viable. He suggested that I continue bed rest, getting up only to use the restroom. At least I could chuck the bed pan!

After reading Dr. Travers's report, Dr. Jackman, with a perplexed look on her face, decided to send me home. I wasn't sure if that was the right call, but I didn't argue.

Returning home, I noticed right away that something was amiss. The tension in the air was suffocating. Later, when I got up to use the restroom, I could hear angry voices through the wall. I returned to the couch. My grandmother was crying. I called for my mom, and asked her what was going on, and she blew it off, saying that my grandmother was just overwhelmed. I knew that there was more to the story. It was clear to me that my situation had caused so much stress that people were starting to fall apart and turn on one another. Hopelessness consumed me.

Around 4 am, I was awakened by another bleeding episode. Although I was lying still and completely horizontal, the blood aggressively spouted out of me. I awakened James who again rushed me to the hospital.

After going through the familiar ritual of questions and tests, the doctor on duty flashed the same bewildered look that we had been seeing for weeks now.

"It seems that these bleeding episodes are increasing in frequency. You were just here yesterday. I'm not sure why you were released so quickly. But in either case, it doesn't make sense for us to admit you, release you, and then re-admit you on a daily basis. I think that our best option is to admit you to Stanford for the remainder of the pregnancy. That way the Stanford doctors that you've been seeing upstairs can take over your care completely. I recommend that you go upstairs for another ultrasound – Dr. Al-Fayadh is on duty today – and then we can get the ball rolling to transfer you to Stanford."

As much as I hated the separation from my children, I knew that Dr. Hicks was right. I needed to stay in the hospital. I didn't see the point however, in going upstairs for yet another ultrasound. I just had an ultrasound the previous day. Each time I saw Ellie's face it tore me to pieces. I became more attached to her, more terrified at what she would have to face as things deteriorated. I was also not enthusiastic about another meeting with Dr. Al-Fayadh. He was the one who was aggressively pushing for me to terminate the pregnancy. I told Dr. Hicks what I was thinking. She then had the nerve to suggest that my reservations about seeing Dr. Al-Fayadh had something to do with his ethnicity! If I weren't so exhausted, I would have taken more offense. But I had no energy to defend my principles. All I cared about at this point was protecting Ellie and holding on to my sanity. I assured Dr. Hicks that Dr. Al-Fayadh's ethnicity had not at any point even entered my mind and then let her continue. She went on to explain that she needed Dr. Al-Fayadh's OK for me to be able to transfer to Stanford. So another ultrasound was unavoidable. Fine. Whatever.

After the obligatory ultrasound, Dr. Al-Fayadh brought us into his office. My large wheelchair didn't allow enough space to be able to close the door to the small office. So the doctor left the door slightly open and spoke in a soft voice to preserve our privacy. He spoke slowly, eyes wide, his voice carrying more than enough intensity to compensate for the lack of volume.

"Julie, this is getting really dangerous. The bleeding is increasing. You are anemic, and your platelets are low. We can admit you to Stanford, but no matter where you are, the longer we wait to do something, the more risk there is to your life. We can safely terminate now, but soon that will not be an option."

I could feel myself getting weaker with each passing day, but hearing it so bluntly stated was chilling. I didn't want to die. But still, I wasn't ready to give up on Ellie. I was 21 weeks along. If I could only make it three more, she would have a chance of surviving. I questioned the doctor, "But isn't there is a chance that the bleeding could just stop?"

"We can't predict what will happen with 100% certainty, but we don't have any reason to believe that it will stop. The hematoma is getting larger, and the bleeding episodes are becoming more frequent."

If there were even the slightest chance for Ellie to survive, then I was going to take it. "I'd like to give it at least one more week to see if things improve."

"OK, fair enough," the doctor wearily responded.

That evening I was taken by ambulance to Stanford. My gurney was brought to a large waiting area where scores of other patients also waited in beds that were lined up across one long room. My impression was that this was an area for patients who had come in through the Emergency Room and were waiting to be admitted to the hospital. I was told that there was no available room for me in Maternity at this point, so I would be stuck here until the situation changed. Why didn't they just let me wait in my nice, private room at El Camino Hospital until a vacancy opened up at Stanford?

As James and I waited, we were visited by the resident on duty who drew a thin curtain to separate me from my neighbor. She asked a few questions and performed yet another pelvic exam. The perinatologist on duty also came by to introduce herself. She was soft-spoken and kind. I noticed on her badge that her name was Natalie. How I missed my Natalie!

Time dragged on since there was nothing but the occasional eavesdrop on our neighbors to occupy our minds between the visits with various nurses and doctors. At some point in the evening, we learned from the conversation one bed over that Barack Obama had been elected President of the United States. I normally would have followed the election with great passion, but in my overloaded state, the news may as well have been a weather report. At another point, a woman came in who was in labor with twins. They set her gurney right next to mine, so for many hours, I heard the excitement at every contraction. It wasn't long ago that I was realistically anticipating the experience of delivering twins. Then I was down to one baby. Now one was becoming less likely. I was relieved when the panting Mama-To-Be was finally wheeled off to the delivery room.

Late that night, a resident from neonatology came to visit us, presumably to talk about the processes in the Neonatal Intensive Care Unit. If Ellie made it into the world at all, it was certain that she would be spending time in the NICU. As soon as the doctor said a few sentences, though, I knew that his goals for the conversation did not match mine.

"I want to give you a realistic vision of what to expect." The young, Asian doctor spoke with a grim expression. "If your baby is born earlier than 24 weeks, there is such little chance of survival that we do not make any attempt at resuscitation. After 24 weeks, we do resuscitate babies, but the outcomes are generally very poor. At 24 weeks, half of the babies die shortly after birth. Of the group that does survive, half of those will have serious brain damage and will not be able to live a normal life. They may be deaf, blind, mentally retarded, or virtually vegetative. The other half who do not suffer obvious brain damage will likely encounter problems as they get older, such as learning disabilities, autism, or psychological problems. Our technology has improved over the years, and we are able to save some, but human babies just aren't supposed to be born that early. With each passing week, the odds will get better, but still serious complications are very likely until we get to around 32 weeks. Now I understand that there is a huge hematoma on your placenta. Having a compromised placenta may have already done damage to your baby's brain development that we can't see. Plus as the hematoma and the baby both get larger, the baby will not have room to move around and will develop physical problems due to the limited motion. I just want to make sure that you have all of the facts as you make decisions in the coming weeks. Do you have any questions?"

James and I sat stunned. We probably asked some questions. But all I can remember is the sinking. Deeper down with each movement of the doctor's lips. Deeper still with each movement of the child on borrowed time inside of me. Ever since the complications started, I had held up 24 weeks as the magical threshold over which Ellie would have a fighting chance for survival. But I had never pictured what *survival* actually meant. If by some miracle, I did manage not to die by 24 weeks, and I delivered Ellie, both she and I would likely die in the process. If she survived in some kind of a vegetative state, what would happen to my family? James would be a widower with four children, two of whom already had special needs, and one that would require round-the-clock care for her entire life. But this scenario was based on even making it to 24 weeks. If I continued to bleed as I had been, there would be no way to make it there anyway. If I continued like this, we would both die. What was my responsibility to Ellie? What was my responsibility to my family that I already had? And why the hell was I being forced to make this kind of totally jacked-up decision? Could life have possibly dealt more cruel a scenario?

My mind thrashed for the next few hours until around midnight, the nurse informed us that my room was finally ready. As I scooted from gurney to bed, I realized how truly dizzy and weak I was. My skin was blotchy. In that instant, the awareness hit me that I *was* actually dying.

Throughout that night, I passed back and forth between nightmare and conscious thought, two indistinguishable monsters. By morning, I had come to a decision of sorts. If I were to receive any sign that I would be able to survive for three more weeks, I would keep going and deliver my baby no matter what the risk to me. But if my condition continued to worsen, I would not allow both of us to die. I decided to broach the subject with James to hear his views. We would need to be clear on what we wanted, especially if it got to the point at which I became incapable of making the call myself.

"Sweetie," I said as I took his hand. My throat tightened. I had no idea how to form the words which I wanted to say. There were no words which I wanted to say. "We have to agree on how far we are willing to go before…" I took a shaky breath. I wasn't getting any further.

"I understand," James responded, his face braced as for a brutal punch.

"If the bleeding gets worse," I continued, "And it is clear that we won't make it to 24 weeks, I can't abandon our kids."

"No," James' red eyes winced, "I don't know what I would do if I lost you. We all need you." His jaw clenched tightly. "Why is this happening to us? This is so unfair!" He buried his face in my shoulder.

From that point on, I never stopped crying. I went on with the motions of life – brushing my teeth, eating breakfast, turning on the television – and my tears continued their mass evacuation from my sinking-ship body. In the morning, the attending physician came by for rounds with his eager team of young interns. In hushed tones, the doctor briefed his students on my status, commenting that my platelets had taken another drop due to the internal bleeding.

At midday, James left my bedside to get some lunch. Minutes after he left, it happened. The blood came out with such force that I could actually hear the gush. I called the nurse. She came in and pulled my covers off. She could not hide her shock as she saw the pool of blood that was forming on the bed. She paged the doctor. People came running in.

"You have to call my husband! Please, call my husband!" I shouted as a crowd gathered around me. A nurse pulled out a Doppler and started looking for a heartbeat. *Why torture me with that? I know she is still alive. I know she will not be soon.* The team propped me up on an upside-down bed pan with a towel over it, and a resident performed a pelvic exam. Everything was so raw inside that the speculum may as well have been a knife. My body shook uncontrollably as the doctor examined me. She quickly determined that my cervix was closed, and again, I was not going into labor. As she withdrew the speculum, softball-sized clots came out with it. The team exchanged looks of horror. I continued to shiver.

James came in amid the commotion. A perplexed phlebotomist scratched his head as he searched for a vein which hadn't already been pricked for blood tests or IV lines. On the third or fourth prick, he finally found a working vein and drained some more of the now precious commodity. James asked the frenzied staff if anyone had taken my blood pressure. Someone ran out for the blood pressure equipment.

Blood continued to empty out of my body with no reduction in the velocity. "It's still coming out so fast!" I frantically told the nurses. I don't know what I expected anyone to do about it. It wasn't as if they could just put a cork in me. There was only one way to stop the bleeding, and no one in the room wanted to be the one to say it.

As life violently drained, I realized that this was the moment James and I had discussed. The revolting moment in which it became clear that Ellie and I would both die if immediate action were not taken. Two mothers inside of me were battling for survival. Marsha, Jesse, and Natalie's mom, desperate to be there for her living children, hung haphazardly over the vast abyss, her fingers tightly gripping the cliff-side. Ellie's mom angrily attacked the shameful, hanging woman, aiming all of her strength toward prying off each pathetic finger, one by one. What kind of a mother would consider murdering her own, innocent baby - the precious girl that was still kicking away inside? This disgraceful woman didn't deserve to live at the expense of her child. The hanging mother didn't have any strength to fight or think or even cry out, but nonetheless, her hands held fast. Ellie's mom knew full well that Ellie had no chance to live at this point no matter what she did, even if she succeeded at prying off the tenth clinging finger. But she didn't care. She stopped prying and started beating her fists against the demon hands. She pounded until her strength was gone, but the weaker woman did not loosen her grip. Ellie's mother fell to the floor, writhing in pain as I spoke, and the bustling room became suddenly quiet.

"I think it's time that we discuss," Those were the only words that my weak voice could get out. I looked at James.

"Termination." James had to be the one to say the fowl word which completed my sentence.

Upon hearing the word, the visibly relieved resident who was caring for me said, "It's the only thing you can do."

My request for a discussion was immediately considered to be a decision. The staff made a sudden transition from befuddled mode to action mode. A surgeon was paged and an operating room was scheduled. I was informed that I would be lucky enough to have the top surgeon in the nation at performing the D&E procedure that I was about to undergo. Probably my uterus would come through unscathed, and I would be able to get pregnant again. *Why the hell would I ever get pregnant again? I don't care what happens to that cursed, useless organ. Take it out and kick it across the room for all I care.*

James took the resident aside for a moment. When they returned, both pairs of eyes were moist and red. James knelt at my bedside.

"The doctor said that Ellie won't feel any pain during the procedure." He could barely speak. "The anesthesia that they give you will also go to her." We sobbed together as the team raced around us. Ellie continued to stir as if nothing were going on.

The nurse brought a pill. I was instructed to place it in my cheek and let it dissolve. It was intended to soften and open the cervix. I remembered a similar pill which I had taken before my first D&C and the pain that it had initiated. All I wanted at this point was to be sedated. I didn't want to feel anything. Now that the vile decision had been made, I wanted to melt into numbness. I asked for a sedative, and the doctor agreed.

Unfortunately, the morphine had no effect, and as soon as the pill in my mouth dissolved, my uterus contracted and did not let go, even for a second. The pain was so intense that it actually came within inches of trumping the emotional pain. I thrashed about in that state for three hours before the mask containing the general anesthesia was finally mercifully placed over my mouth. Three words played in a loop as I drifted off. *I'm so sorry. I'm so sorry.*

"Julie," A voice pulled me from the darkness. I kept my eyes shut. *Please, just let me be with her on the other side.* "Julie." The voice was persistent. I slowly opened my eyes to see a nurse standing over me. The first thing that I noticed was my vacant pelvis. There was nothing. No bleeding, no pain, no movement. Everything I knew was gone.

"You came through just fine." The voice said, "You just need to stay here while we get a bit of blood into you." I glanced over at my stinging hand to see blood flowing into my IV.

The Descent

I nodded and reclosed my eyes, seeking rescue from the excruciating calm of my body. Sleep cradled my broken heart in its gentle arms. All I wanted was to stay there forever.

I fought consciousness with all of my might, but eventually, I had to wake up. As James saw my eyes open, he wrapped me in his arms. We held each other and cried. This was a new level of sadness that I had never touched before. It was as if every cell in my body had been tinted dark gray. I unwillingly existed. Inexplicably, my heart beat, my lungs expanded and contracted, but there was nothing alive inside.

The hospital staff avoided me. This worked well as I preferred being left alone. My sole visitor was a social worker who came by and gave me a folder full of resources for psychological counseling and support groups which I fully intended to chuck in the garbage. Who could possibly even come close to understanding this?

At one point, a resident called me on my bedside phone. He asked how I was doing. I said fine. He said that he would go ahead and release me from the hospital. I found it strange that no doctor was even going to examine me or give me any instructions before sending me home, but I didn't care. I wasn't eager to stay in the hospital or eager to go home. What difference did any of it make?

The nurse came by to wheel me out to the car. She pushed my chair out the door, stopped abruptly, and made a swift U-turn back into the room.

"Oh, just a minute," she said with a flustered look. She wandered out to the hall, leaving my door open a crack. I peeked through the crack, and realized the reason for her nervous stalling. Right at that moment, another woman was being triumphantly wheeled out to her car, baby in arms.

"There, we're ready now," the nurse said as she returned to the room and resumed my exit from Maternity. We met James at the car and the two of us headed home. I didn't want to see anyone, not even my children. I just wanted to disappear under the covers of my bed. I slept. I woke up. I cried. I slept. Inside of me, not a soul kicked.

Chapter 36
Ellie's Milk

On my first trip to the restroom after returning home, I assessed the state of my body. I was slightly dizzy, slightly weak - an appalling contrast to my withering state only one day ago. My body felt despicably normal. I was angered by how quickly and callously it could move on now that its tiny occupant had been evicted. It just didn't seem right.

The other thing I began to notice was that my breasts were enlarged, sore, and hard as rocks. On my shirt two little wet blotches were emerging. My milk, or more accurately, Ellie's milk had come in.

Taking my first shower in a month, I tried to shield my tender breasts from the hot water. *This is not how it was supposed to be – the milk that I was dying to feed you drying up inside.* As I shampooed my hair, a stirring in my abdomen interrupted my thoughts. A flicker of excitement burst out of the ashes - had the doctor accidentally left Ellie inside? I lingered for an instant in delusion before my intellect dragged me back to empty reality. The steamy water swept more tears down the drain. It felt good to scrub the weeks of scum off of me, but at the same time, I found it unbearable to spend so much one-on-one time with the body which had failed me so miserably. My belly was still quite enlarged, but it no longer had the healthy plumpness that had filled my maternity shirts. Now it was more like an overripe fruit, plucked from the vine and left to the elements. I half expected flies to be attracted to its rot. I glanced down at my swollen breasts which never got the message that there was no Ellie to feed. Ironically, they were the one part of my body that was actually doing its job. Little good that did.

I paused. Maybe there *was* something to salvage here. Another shower idea started swirling around in my brain. Maybe my one functioning reproductive bit could actually serve a purpose. After all, I did have a baby. Natalie was only 13 months old, and she was quite scrawny. What if I fed her Ellie's milk? She could at least get some benefit of breast milk. For the first time since Ellie's death, the mother in me opened her bloodshot eyes. She was still groggy and listless, but no longer dead asleep.

I mentioned the idea to my mother later that day. She dropped everything and raced to the store to buy a breast pump. Within an hour, she had it sterilized and set up for me. I gave it a go, staring at the empty bottle as the pump unnaturally contorted my painful nipple. As time passed and the bottle remained empty, I wondered if I had been too quick to assume that any part of my body could actually function properly. Just as I was ready to give up and declare my womanhood a complete waste of X chromosomes, a couple of small drops landed in the bottle. Then a couple more. After pumping both breasts, I victoriously beheld one ounce of yellowish liquid which I assumed must be collostrum.

I wondered if Natalie would totally reject it, since she had never tasted breast milk. I thought about mixing it with regular milk and gradually getting her used to the flavor. But ultimately, I decided to feed it to her straight to see what she would think of it.

As Natalie relaxed into my lap, her body melted into mine. This was the feeling that I had tried so hard to forget while my arms laid empty in my hospital bed. Breathing Natalie in, I felt like a freed prisoner of war taking the first sniff of a warm, inviting post-rescue meal. For the first time since returning to my house, I was home. Natalie's fingers stroked the sides of the bottle as she began to drink. I braced myself for her response to this foreign beverage.

Natalie had always been a highly lackadaisical eater. A single ounce of milk could take her a full five minutes to consume. This time though, she guzzled the bottle down in a

The Pursuit of Family

series of powerful gulps. She withdrew the bottle, smiled at me, and said, "Mo pwease."

By this point, James and I had poured six years of tireless effort into our goal to sustain a successful pregnancy. Not only had the goal never been reached, but the fallout left behind was devastating. We were in debt up to our ears. Our one biological baby who survived past the first trimester never got to experience life outside of the womb for even one second. Our adopted children were neglected and traumatized. Our entire family was in a state of raw shock. The stress that these years had inflicted on James and me must have shaved decades off of our lives. We were weary and empty, with far more than our chronological share of deep cry-lines and gray hairs. Until this moment, there had not been a single positive outcome resulting from our infertility struggle. With Natalie's acceptance and enjoyment of the milk, we could place one small item on the positive side of the balance, whose massive negative side was causing the floor beneath it to buckle. Natalie would benefit from the nutritious milk, filled with protective antibodies. And I would get to retain at least a partial experience of one of the aspects of biological motherhood. I would nourish my child with my milk. Not that this small victory came anywhere close to making even a fraction of the struggle worthwhile. But at least we didn't walk away with nothing.

Chapter 37
Throbbing

As time passed, my wounds throbbed in slow motion. There were moments when I would be outside with my children, and a breathtakingly blue sky would wrap me in a soft, amnesiac blanket. My breathing would deepen, and I would experience a momentary peace.

Interspersed with these moments were times when my inner storm would have full authority over my consciousness. I would be with my children and be objectively aware that the cuteness of their actions was reaching mind-blowing levels. However, the chip inside of me which revels and appreciates, would be completely disabled. I would feel absolutely nothing. These moments terrified me.

Early-on in my recovery, I started having panic attacks, often striking in the middle of the night. The stress during the pregnancy that I had fended off with books and other distractions in order to protect the baby had never gone away. My tactics had only served to delay facing the tucked-away demons. Now they were organizing and attacking during quiet moments when my defenses were down. I would break out in a cold sweat, my heart racing, and ramblings of death and nothingness would fill my head. One night, the insomnia absolutely would not relent. By 2:00 am, I was completely frantic. I didn't want to disturb James. If I leaned on him any more than I already was, he wouldn't be able to support his own weight. But I felt like if I didn't talk to someone, I would be fitted for a straight jacket before sunup. I decided to call my mother. My call's harsh interruption of her sleep undoubtedly initiated her own mini panic attack, but she answered with a calm voice as if I had called to shoot the breeze at two in the afternoon. She talked with me and listened to me rant for at least an hour, until I finally wound down and became sleepy. I returned to bed, and slept well with the certainty that beneath my shaky, clumsy tight-rope walk, my family stood, net firmly in hand.

There is nothing that rivals the power of children to keep one's thoughts in the here and now. Rushing to various appointments, breaking up bitter disputes over toys, feeding, bathing, reading stories, and tidying the messes that followed them as tightly as their shadows, I had very little time to dwell on grief. This was both good and bad. My life had no choice but to move on, and the more I was present with my children, the happier I felt. But sometimes I wished that I could just take a break or maybe even a short trip like we had done in the grieving days before Jesse. It was both physically and psychologically exhausting trying to keep up with two toddlers.

I found that grief would always catch me by surprise. One day I decided that it was time to face the rotting wasteland of my refrigerator, which had not been cleaned out since my pre-bed rest days. I expected the experience to be disgusting and possibly vomit-inducing, but I didn't anticipate the emotional impact. Each of the recognizable food items assaulted me with one flash back or another. I came across a container of pineapple, half devoured by what looked like multiple species of mold. I remembered the day I had happily eaten that pineapple during a visit with James' brother only days before Dr. Fisher pronounced that Ellie would soon be dead. He had been surprised to see how pregnant I was looking. We sat and ate, and the world was a happy place. My desperate time machine fantasy kicked off again. Maybe if I could just go back to that perfect pineapple day, I could do something different that could have prevented the disaster. Maybe I could go back to that time and feel the ignorant hope kicking away inside of me just one more time.

The next meal I recognized dragged me on another journey. It was the mock ravioli that my mom had cooked for me at one point while I was on bed rest. The mere sight of the food sent me right back to the family room couch, lying on my side, awkwardly spooning the food into my mouth. Feeding an aching, grimy body that was in the process of failing me once again. This second living of the moment did not dilute the agony in the least. I wished that the mold could eat away at the memories until they were barely recognizable. It was bad enough living through it once.

Another constant reminder hung in my closet and taunted me at every opportunity. My maternity clothes, which I had so blissfully prepared, had transformed into a constant source of torture. I didn't want to have to keep seeing them, but I didn't want to face putting them away for good. Practicality eventually won the battle. I would need some clothes to wear besides the handful of sweats that I had spent the past month in. Somehow, my pre-pregnancy wardrobe would have to return to my closet. Finally, I asked James to bring the boxes of my clothes back in from the garage. He brought the clothing in and placed it on the floor in our bedroom.

Seeing the pain on my face, James took hold of my hands. "Why don't I pack the maternity clothes, and you can hang the old ones back up. I don't know where anything goes."

I wrapped my arms around him. "I can't stop crying," I said.

"You don't need to stop crying," he replied holding me tightly, "It's OK. Just let it out."

So I took his advice. James put on some music, and we worked away side by side. Both sets of clothing soaked up the tears that the tissues weren't quick enough to catch. When it was over and everything was put away, I was completely exhausted, but I did feel immense relief that it was done. With a little help from my husband, I had faced a demon and survived. I had stolen back a fraction of life's power to jerk me around.

My re-matriculation into society was exponentially more difficult than it had been after past miscarriages. This time, every person who had seen my belly over the past couple of months knew that I had been pregnant. Some knew what had happened, but others were left to wonder. When I returned to my previous activities, I felt so many stares as people scanned my body for the mysteriously missing pregnancy bump.

Each time I saw someone for the first time, it was awkward and stressful. People squirmed as they had in the past, not knowing what to say or do to help. I mostly just redirected conversations and tried to take the focus off of me. Each time I checked someone off of the *haven't seen since pregnant* list, I began to notice a faint feeling of empowerment.

I returned to work two weeks before my medical leave was up so that I could get the final set of initial encounters over with. I still made frequent escapes to the restroom for crying sessions, but I was incrementally reclaiming my life. By Christmas, my encounters with people were mostly normal. My grief and loss still sat like nettle on my heart, but at least they weren't paraded out any more for the whole world to see.

In February, Marsha went on a school trip to Japan. While she was gone, I decided to organize her very messy room and surprise her with her own computer. I started my search for a computer desk at the local Salvation Army, hoping to get lucky and find a bargain. On my way there, I felt a surge of excitement. It felt good to be doing something special for my Marsha. It felt good to once again have the strength to be a mother. As I stopped at a red light, I noticed a group of people gathered on the sidewalk right in front of me. They were holding up signs of protest. As my mind made the connection that they were standing in front of a Planned Parenthood building, I realized what it was that they were protesting. One of them hoisted up a poster-sized image of a dismembered, presumably aborted baby. I should have turned away, but I couldn't pull my eyes off of the image. Was that my Ellie? Had some employee of the hospital secretly taken a picture of her and blown it up to show the world the gruesome manner in which she died? I had only seen her in fuzzy ultrasound pictures, so for all I knew, that could have been her. Was that what she looked like when the lights were turned off in the operating room the day that she so violently left my body?

I silently pleaded with the baby in the picture.

If you take one thing from this world, let it be the understanding that your parents loved you and wanted you more than anything.

The picture blurred as my eyes filled with tears.

Please understand that we would have done anything if there had been a chance to save you. Not a day goes by that I don't wish that I could have gone with you and that you didn't have to leave this world all alone.

I couldn't stand to look any longer. I turned my eyes to the crowd of people. They all proudly stood, holding their signs, basking in their righteousness. I knew that they all believed in what they were doing, but couldn't they have made their point without exploiting that poor baby? Now her only appearance before the world would be in her moment of greatest indignity. Now onlookers would accept the lie that she was some sort of inconvenience to her parents that some evil doctor helped them to get rid of. I knew differently. She was a beautiful, strong girl who brought her family immeasurable joy despite the far too short period of her existence. Whether or not that baby was Ellie, she was someone's beloved child. That is how she should be remembered. I was certain that not a single one of the protesters were ever faced with that kind of a horrendously impossible choice, to live without their daughter or to die with her. Yet there they stood, telling me that they wanted me dead. I thought back to the recent presidential debates when John McCain discussed late term abortion to save the mother's life, flippantly wrapping in air quotes the words *women's health.* How dare he wrap the anguish of my husband losing his wife, my children losing their mother within a gesture reserved only for sarcasm? Only someone who has been through this hell can even attain an inkling of understanding of how it feels to have a moving, breathing part of you sliced out of your body against your will, but by your choice. It is this kind of insensitivity that continually assaults victims of infertility. No one understands.

I remembered suddenly that my children were also in the car. They had experienced enough trauma as it was. They didn't need to be frightened by an image of a mutilated baby. I pointed out a balloon I saw on the other side of the street. When the light turned green, I sped away, reminding myself to never drive by that place again. That day, I went home with the last thing that I wanted - an indelible image of my baby's last moments burned into my brain. I didn't find a computer desk at the Salvation Army. I should have just stayed in bed.

Chapter 38
Babies on Ice

As time went on, my worries gradually shifted from the terrifying flashbacks of the trauma to the troubling questions of the future. James and I still had six frozen embryos from our calamitous IVF attempt, and we would eventually have to decide what we were going to do with them. Obviously with no more insight into what happened in the previous pregnancy, it would be reckless to try for another one. The one option we had left which could provide us some information was to have the pregnancy tissue examined. Dr. Brewer's clinic had a pathology lab which was able to analyze pregnancy tissue to pinpoint the immunological issues of the pregnancy. So we sent slides to Dr. Brewer's lab hoping that they would solve the mystery.

When the results were in, I met with Dr. Trober, who wore the perplexed expression typical of doctors in my vicinity. The tissue showed nothing atypical for second trimester pregnancy tissue. There were no uterine NK cells as had been expected - absolutely nothing to explain what had gone wrong. Dr. Trober felt strongly that the problem had an immune etiology, which was why the IVIG treatments seemed to help. However, it was clearly not one of the immune issues that had ever been researched. If I were to try for another pregnancy, he recommended continuing IVIG until the third trimester and adding a steroid called dexamethazone. But he also cautioned that since we didn't really know what was wrong, there would be no guarantee that the treatments would make any difference.

I left the clinic more conflicted than ever. I knew that my family could not survive the stress of another pregnancy.

And given what happened last time, I couldn't guarantee my own physical survival of another pregnancy. But then what were we to do with our embryos? We had a responsibility toward them now that we'd created them. Throwing them away was not an option. And I couldn't see us donating them to another couple when our family was not yet complete. I figured the only option was to wait. Maybe in five to ten years, someone might make a breakthrough and figure out what my problem was. My age would be less of a factor since the embryos were created with 32 year old eggs. I'd heard in the news about women over 60 carrying pregnancies to term when the eggs were donated by younger women.

But how could I survive more years with this unresolved? I knew myself well enough to be sure that the tiny flicker of hope would constantly taunt me and prevent me from moving on with my life. Part of me kept thinking about how close we had come with Ellie. Maybe if I had not stopped the IVIG at 12 weeks, she would have never had any problems. Maybe I could just give it one more try and everything would just magically be different. But the smarter part of me knew that whether or not it would work, we couldn't risk our family's well-being any more for this dream. I had to find a way to close the book on this and start accepting my life as it was. Barring some ridiculous miracle, I would never experience a successful pregnancy, and we would never have a biological child, no matter how much I wanted it to happen.

It was right about that time that everything changed, when a friend approached James with a surprising suggestion. James and I had both known Tanisha for many years on a casual basis. She knew about our situation and really felt for us. Having five healthy children of her own, she absolutely loved being pregnant, but did not want any more children. She had always dreamed of helping a family which was not blessed with her incredible fertility. She told James that if we were interested, she would like to carry our child for us. James was blown away by this sudden, generous gesture. He thanked her for the offer and told her that we would keep it in mind as we tried to figure out the next step.

When James told me about the encounter, I immediately flashed back to my high school days, when I had promised my two best friends that if they couldn't have children, I would love to be their surrogate. They both had health issues which could have prevented them from becoming mothers. However, both ended up producing lovely children and would not be requiring my services, though with the baby in me, I wouldn't really call it a service. Irony sucks.

James and I decided to wait a while before making any decisions. We needed to get ourselves and our family back on track before pursuing yet another potentially disastrous avenue. We let several months pass, and when we felt strong enough, we set out to learn more about surrogacy. I called around and found out what the requirements, costs, and processes were for a surrogacy. It looked like the legal fees, surrogate screening fees, and medical costs amounted to around $12,000. This was actually less than I had expected. Since we already had the embryos, we wouldn't have to pay for a fresh IVF cycle, so that saved us a significant amount. I had no idea what kind of fee Tanisha would want. Typically the surrogate's fee is the bulk of the cost.

As daunting as the thought of throwing more money toward another potentially losing battle was, it was actually the lengthy process that overwhelmed me the most. First Tanisha would be medically screened. Then Tanisha, her husband, James and I would all undergo psychological evaluation. Next we would work with our respective attorneys (all of whom James and I would be paying for) to hammer out a legal contract. I found out that we did have one bit of good fortune, as California is one of the kindest states toward surrogacy. In some states, surrogacy is prohibited by law. In others, the surrogate is considered the legal parent until she actually gives the child up to be adopted by the biological parents at birth. Luckily California is one of the states in which the concept of a pre-birth order exists. This order is signed around five months into the pregnancy, and it declares the biological parents as the legal parents. When the child is born, the biological parents assume legal rights to the baby, and their names appear on the birth certificate from the start.

Once the contract is signed, the intense medical portion begins. Tanisha would go on the birth control pill, followed by subcutaneous Lupron injections for 3-3.5 weeks. During that time, she would be taking prenatal vitamins, baby aspirin, dexamethizone (a steroid), and antibiotics. Upon starting the cycle, Tanisha would begin intramuscular estradial injections two times per week, until the tenth week of pregnancy. Near the time of the transfer, she would start daily intramuscular progesterone shots, which she would also continue until the tenth week of pregnancy. In addition to the progesterone shots, she would take progesterone suppositories until the 12th week of pregnancy. Except for the estradial injections, I had experienced all of those medications with my IVF cycle, and I could not imagine someone putting their body through all of that for me. With all of these treatments, there was still only a 30-40% likelihood of Tanisha becoming pregnant in a given frozen embryo cycle. So potentially, she could have to do many cycles of shots before finally achieving pregnancy. It had been a lovely thought, but once Tanisha sensed the enormity of this process, she would back out. And I still wasn't sure if I wanted to do this myself.

James and I discussed it and decided to contact her anyway and keep an open mind. I arranged to meet Tanisha for lunch. I prepared a list of questions for her and brought my notes from the research that I had done. As prepared as I was, I still felt like I had no clue what I was doing. What is the etiquette for meeting with the woman who has offered to carry your child?

When I arrived at the restaurant, Tanisha was already there. She sat tall yet relaxed. When she saw me, she smiled and we started shooting the breeze like old friends. I felt more at ease with each moment I spent with her. Tanisha spoke about how she had always wanted to do this for someone. She had had five easy and uncomplicated pregnancies, and thoroughly enjoyed being pregnant. She felt she was psychologically prepared and that she would not feel any attachment to the baby. She had thought through how she would explain the pregnancy to her children, sensing that she would have to be very careful with her second-to-youngest daughter to reiterate that the baby wouldn't be coming home to their house. She had researched on the internet to find stories of other surrogates to find out what the experience was like. This was clearly not an impulsive whim for Tanisha. I strongly sensed her true passion for this endeavor, and it was obvious that she had thought it out extensively. She also didn't give off the vibe that she was making a huge personal sacrifice so that she could be perceived as some sort of a savior. She seemed genuinely excited about the experience and played down her own generosity and sacrifice.

Then I dropped the bomb of all of my research. I described in detail the intrusive screening, the painful shots, the mind boggling cocktail of medications that she would be subjecting her body to. She bit her lip and winced as I graphically and brutally described what it would be like from first-hand experience.

She took a deep breath and said, "I think I can handle it. You said the shots are only for 12 weeks, right?" She sat straighter, and her eyes filled with resolve. "I'd be fine with that."

Her determination had not wavered even for a second. She not only was willing, but she really wanted to do this. I braced myself for the last question which had been hiding under my tongue for the entire encounter, waiting for an ideal moment to emerge, all the while knowing there would be none.

"What are your expectations when it comes to the fee?"

Tanisha was not a wealthy woman. She was still finishing up her bachelor's degree while working full time and raising five young children. She had college loans which she would be surely be paying back for many years to come. I would have understood if she had wanted to benefit financially from this arrangement. Who wouldn't take an opportunity to gain financial stability for their family? However, I knew that along with all of the other expenses of a surrogacy, James and I simply could not afford to pay a standard surrogate fee, which ranged from $20,000 - $40,000. We were already deep in the hole from the previous years of infertility-induced financial drain.

Tanisha did not hesitate to answer, "I don't feel that it's morally right to ask for a fee for something like this. This is something that I want to do for you, not for the money. I'll leave that part up to you and James."

I was so impressed by everything about Tanisha. It seemed to me that if our baby could not gestate in me, then I could not ask for a better substitute. Another thing that occurred to me was that if I kept pumping milk for Natalie, I could actually nurse a baby despite not carrying it. That way, I could approach a small step closer to the towering asymptote which separated me from the natural experience of motherhood. I still wasn't sure about how I felt about turning over the pregnancy to someone else, but I did feel a high level of confidence in Tanisha's good motives and her ability to carry it through. We decided to meet again with our respective husbands to discuss it further.

Meeting Tanisha and her husband, Orlando, for dinner to discuss the surrogacy was the strangest double date I have ever been on. James and I had met Orlando before in passing, but had never actually talked with him. We had no idea what to expect. I imagined that the average husband would not be thrilled at the thought of his wife carrying another couple's child for nine long months.

Contrary to our fears, Orlando was warm and friendly right from the start. The four of us got along beautifully. The conversation was effortless, and we found that we all had a lot in common. We talked at length about children, politics, travel, food, even religion. Every topic imaginable - except for surrogacy. It went on like this for over an hour. When all of our plates were empty and there was a lull in the conversation, Tanisha finally had the guts to point out the hefty, yet silent pachyderm perched on the table that we were all skillfully dancing around. Once the topic was finally opened, we each spoke about our feelings and expectations. James and I described our past experiences with pregnancy and conveyed how grateful we were that Tanisha was considering this. Tanisha reiterated her confidence in her ability and willingness to do this. Orlando said that he had been concerned that Tanisha might have a hard time giving up a baby that she'd carried for nine months. In addition to her psychological health, he worried about her physical health, especially if she became pregnant with twins. He told us that he had discussed his concerns with her, and that she still felt certain that she was up for it. That was enough for him to decide that he would support her in whatever she chose to do. Looking at her with pure admiration, he stated that there was no better person in the world to do this for us. He said that he felt with 100% certainty that if we went through with this, we would end up with a baby.

The four of us left, agreeing that we would go through the initial screening to see if this would even be a possibility. It was hard to know how to feel. James and I were experiencing a rip-roaring tug of war between excitement and hesitance. The deeper we got into this, the further the concept was moving out of safe theoretical space. This really could happen. We just had to make absolutely sure, before we got too far in, that we actually wanted it to happen.

The more the surrogacy process got rolling, the more momentum it gained. Before we knew it, the medical screening was complete, and Tanisha had been given the green light. Next came the psychological evaluation. The lawyer which the clinic recommended was also a licensed marriage and family counselor, so she was able to do the psychological screening of all four of us. When James and I met with her for our evaluation, it was easy and painless for the most part. The one thing that she did really press us on was the financial aspect. She wanted us to determine an exact figure for what we wanted to pay Tanisha and make sure that it matched with Tanisha's expectations. She said that even though Tanisha had left that up to us, she still had an expectation in her mind of what the figure should be. We had to determine early on if our figure matched with hers, because if it didn't, then it wouldn't be a good match.

The lawyer had also pushed Tanisha to do the same sort of thinking about the fee. She had urged Tanisha to seriously consider the costs to herself and to determine an amount that would make sure there would be no resentment down the line. As it turned out, Tanisha's figure was slightly higher than we expected, though still considerably lower than the standard surrogate fee. Still, it made us stop dead in our tracks. Would we be able to pull this off financially, as totally drained as we were? Panic set in. Were we putting our family in more jeopardy for another attempt that may not succeed? Plus, I still didn't feel ready to let go of carrying the baby myself. We decided to take a few weeks and give careful consideration before making a decision. Tanisha was completely understanding and did not push us at all.

The more I thought about it, the more I convinced myself that I could try just one more time for another pregnancy myself. After all, with the additional medications on board, there was a chance that it could go to term with no problems whatsoever. If it didn't end up working out, then maybe a year from now, we could consider surrogacy with the remaining embryos. The more I thought about it, the more seduced I became by the possibility of having another baby kicking inside of me. The possibility of having a baby the *normal* way. Not having to awkwardly explain to anyone where this new baby who looks kind of like us appeared from all of a sudden. Not having to admit that I simply couldn't do it myself.

I focused all of my energy toward convincing myself and James to do this one final try. One night, James stopped me in the middle of one of my compelling monologues and said,

"But I keep thinking about how I would feel if something bad were to happen to another one of our babies. What if we get a little further this time, but the baby ends up being born with severe disabilities? I don't know if we could forgive ourselves."

The truth in his statement hit me like an errant football to the nose. Part of our job as parents is to make difficult choices and sacrifices to protect our children. I knew that no matter how many treatments I had, there was still no question that the safest place for our baby was inside of Tanisha and not inside of me. It would be morally wrong for me to put my child at risk to satisfy my own selfish dreams when there was a safer alternative available. The clarity of that moment was suffocating.

"You're right." I whispered. "We have to do the right thing for our babies. We need to put them where we know they'll be safest."

James and I held each other as we said another goodbye to the life that we thought we would live. We would never experience the innocent bliss of a normal pregnancy. James would never support his wife as she waddled out to the car, counting the minutes between contractions. We would never hold hands and breathe together through hard labor. We would never experience that moment when my finger nails have worn holes in his hands, and the lusty wailing of our baby cancels out any thought of pain. We would never take that triumphant wheelchair ride to the car with our baby wrapped in my arms. We would be left to watch things like that through cracks in doorways. The decision was made.

Chapter 39
The View from the Sidelines

When I notified Tanisha, she was ecstatic. She couldn't wait to get started and wanted to begin the meds at the start of her next cycle. So we got things moving on the legal contract. That process was easy, since we were in agreement on everything already. Before we knew it, Tanisha was on the medications. Dr. Zoumis recommended that I come along for Tanisha's final ultrasound before the transfer so that we could discuss how many and which embryos we would be transferring.

Driving down Highway 101 on the way to Dr. Zoumis' clinic, I passed one-by-one the off-ramps leading to El Camino Hospital, then Stanford Hospital. The ghosts of doctors and hospitals past flooded my mind. It seemed every place, every smell, every ray of the sun was bursting with memories of hope and loss. My morning allergies had swollen my eyes. I wondered if Tanisha and the staff at the clinic would think that I had been crying. I adjusted my sitting position as the uncomfortable bloating of my ovaries taunted me with an ironic reminder. I was ovulating today. What a joke!

When the nurse called Tanisha in, I stood to go with her, and the nurse stopped me, saying they'd call me when Tanisha was ready. Of course, I realized, it would be better for her to get undressed without me in the room. This made sense, but it punctuated the fact that I was not the person being cared for here. I was an outsider, watching from the sidelines.

When I was called to join Tanisha, I wondered how awkward it would be to sit with her, her legs in the stirrups, a paper sheet barely covering her. Tanisha's demeanor quelled this fear immediately. She sat upright with no sense of embarrassment, her face beaming with the approaching possibility. We started talking about the transfer, and I showed her the details I had jotted down about our frozen embryos. Dr. Zoumis entered the room.

"Good to see you again," he smiled as he shook my hand. "Tanisha, good to see you as well. Are we getting excited?"

Tanisha gave a spirited, "Oh yeah!"

I tried to match her enthusiasm, but my eyes shifted towards the floor as I chimed in with my "Yeah." I remembered the last time I saw Dr. Zoumis, the day that I first cradled my twins inside of me. Here I was slinking back, having destroyed two completely flawless embryos, unfit to house any more of them.

Dr. Zoumis narrated as he performed the ultrasound, delivering high praise of Tanisha's uterine lining. Conditions were perfect in here. This should have made me happy. I was unsure what I was feeling. Dr. Zoumis chatted with us for a bit and recommended transferring two of our normal embryos. He said that on a frozen cycle, the odds of pregnancy when implanting only one embryo would be 20%, which is obviously quite low. Transferring two embryos would up the pregnancy odds to 50%, and if she were to get pregnant, the odds of a singleton pregnancy were 90%. Logically, I agreed that transferring two made sense, but inside I longed to hang on to all of the normal embryos for myself, for some possibility, or more accurately, impossibility, in the future. I felt like I was giving them away.

After Dr. Zoumis left, the nurse went over medications with Tanisha. The nurse kept asking me if I had any questions. Why would I have questions? The meds were not for me anymore.

After the appointment, Tanisha and I stood outside and talked for a bit. I'm not sure exactly what she did, but speaking to her always made me feel OK about things. Not infused with her level of excitement, but OK. Even a little bit excited. The transfer was six days away. When it was my transfer, I couldn't wait for the day to arrive. Now, ambivalence better described my mindset. I wanted it to work. I wanted to have our healthy, beautiful baby. But at the same time, I felt so much less invested in the outcome than I did when it was me. Maybe that was better. Then if she didn't get pregnant, I wouldn't be completely disappointed. A tiny piece of me didn't want a pregnancy to stick and wanted the job reserved only for myself.

On the morning of the transfer, my stomach was in knots. I drove to Tanisha's home to pick her up. Having allowed too much time for getting lost, I arrived ten minutes early. I decided to drive around for a while after locating her address to get myself as centered and calm as possible. However, when I reached Tanisha's house, she was already outside waiting for me, smiling and waving. As soon as she entered the car, we immediately started to chat like we might be a couple of gal pals headed to the mall. This put me more at ease. My comfort with Tanisha was the polar opposite of my discomfort about what was happening today.

As soon as we sat down in Dr. Zoumis' waiting room, my nerves regained their stranglehold. It was a busy day, and there were at least six or seven couples sitting with us. I wondered what they thought of us. Were we lesbian partners, conceiving a baby in the only way possible for us? Were we friends, one of us supporting the other through a procedure? I figured their last guess was that she was going to be my surrogate. Even I had my own mental picture of the kind of woman who would be using a surrogate. I don't know why, but I imagined her as a highly-confident, smartly dressed woman who had bypassed her peak years of fertility by 15 years. With my ragdoll posture, no one would be mistaking me for confident. My "power suit" consisted of jeans, tee-shirt and flip flops. And although I was disturbed by the lines that had surfaced on my face over the past six years, I think they were far less noticeable to others. I was still commonly mistaken for a teenager. It would be a stretch to picture me as a woman who has been at this long enough to have already exhausted every possible fertility option.

The View from the Sidelines

I was the first to be called in to see Dr. Zoumis. He got James on the speaker phone and informed us that both embryos had thawed beautifully. In fact, one of them had even improved its rating by becoming a fully expanded blastocyst after thawing. I flashed back to our IVF, when Dr. Zoumis delivered similar news to us about our now-dead babies. I wished that I could be anywhere else but here. My mind told me that we were doing the right thing, but my heart could not keep pace.

I went in with Tanisha to the procedure room, and I was ushered to a stool in the corner of the room. I felt like I may as well complete the picture by donning a dunce cap. I slumped in the seat, hoping no one would notice my excessive blinking as I tried with all my might to hold back tears. This was the same scene as one year before, only a different lead actress. Watching my embryos, surrendering them to another woman, was like sucking them out of my uterus all over again. I kept trying to remind myself, "This is the safest place for them." But doing the right thing had never been so painful.

Pretty soon, it was over – text-book, successful, irreversible. Now all there was to do was wait.

In the days following the transfer, I noticed one of the perks of surrogacy right away. Since nothing was happening inside of my body, it was much easier to put the whole thing out of my mind and just leave time alone to pass at its own steady pace. Of course the pending news floated through my consciousness regularly, but not at the obsessive level that it would have if I was vigilantly monitoring and safeguarding my own physical state.

Tanisha took her pregnancy test ten days after the transfer. Obsessive worry over the result of the test awakened with my alarm clock that morning, and I could think about nothing else. I wasn't exactly clear on what to worry about because I wasn't sure what I wanted the result to be. Of course, my thinking self wanted it to be successful. If it wasn't, that would mean that more of our babies had silently slipped out of existence. No part of me would ever consciously wish for that to happen. But my feeling, grieving, fundamentally selfish self still longed to escape from having to hear the official confirmation that someone else was going to bear my child for me.

By the afternoon, I was watching the microseconds pass, keeping my cell phone close at hand. Finally at around 4:30 the clinic called with the result. Tanisha was pregnant, and the beta hcg was high. High enough to suspect twins.

"So congratulations," the nurse on the other end said with great excitement, "You're pregnant!" *If only that were true.*

I thanked her for the news. *This is good news. This is good news.* That was my mantra for the day. I figured if I said it enough, the message would spread down to the dark, sad reaches of my consciousness.

This was really happening. And for the first time ever, with me out of the picture, we had an extremely high likelihood of success. I just hoped that if a birth took place eight months from now, it would feel like success.

As sadness had the distinct advantage over all of my other emotions, I realized I needed to do something to get my focus off of the fact that I wasn't the one who was pregnant. I needed to feel more like the mother of this baby (or babies, as the case may be). So I decided to knit a baby blanket. I had bought the yarn and pattern to make for Ellie literally a week before our lives crumbled. So I dug it out of my closet and started the pattern. As each loop passed, one needle to the next, I focused on the little face which would rub against the soft, white moss stitch someday. When we wrapped our baby in this blanket, we would not be thinking about whose uterus had served as incubator. We would just be eternally grateful that he or she was in this world with us. If I could just hold on to that image, maybe I would be able to get through the ensuing months.

Chapter 40
Deja Vu

As our baby was gestating in the next town over, life continued as usual at home. Some days were good, and some were unbearable. It seemed like every small wound I suffered, no matter how unrelated, would reopen the big wound. A bad day with the kids, an argument with James, or even slamming my finger in the car door would bury me beneath the landslide of six years of grief. It was like the scab on Jesse's knee that would just never heal. Each time he fell, the scab would come off, and the wound would gush once again with angry blood. Except in my case, it didn't matter which body part was hit - my scab would pop off. In an instant, I would be back in the hospital swimming in a pool of blood. Back at the moment when I knew that it was really over and I would not be meeting my little girl. Experiencing it again for the first time.

Jesse and Natalie's behavior often knocked off the scab, sending me on an *if only* rampage. I would be overcome by a warped, irrational fantasy that if I had biological children, they would behave perfectly and never cause me undue stress. Logically I knew that this line of thinking was ridiculous and that I would never trade Jesse and Natalie for any other child. But I did feel intense frustration that nothing in life could ever just be easy for me. Sometimes I just was so worn out by it all.

One day, when Jesse and Natalie were having a particularly difficult day, I decided to play a movie and let them chill for a while. I needed to pick something that would fully capture their attention. As I looked, I spotted my wedding video on the shelf. They had never seen it, and I figured they would enjoy pointing out various family members. Sure enough, they were completely captivated. I sat with them on the couch and pointed out people to them. When the vibrant, young bride appeared, it took some convincing to get Jesse to agree that it was me. He said, "That's not you. She has black eyes." I explained to him that I was wearing makeup that day. It struck me that Jesse was right. That wasn't me. I was no longer that young woman, brimming with bliss. I watched her as she spun freely through the wildflowers on highest peak of the most beautiful mountain. There she was, eyes to the heavens, arms outstretched, breathing in the sweet music of life. She had no idea that she was about to be repeatedly struck by lightning.

A couple of hours after the video ended, Jesse said, "I want that Mommy from the movie to come to my house." I smiled. I knew he was probably just referring to the pretty, sparkly get-up. But I couldn't help but agree. I too wished that she would come back.

With each week that passed following the positive pregnancy result, Tanisha got her hormone levels checked, and I got a call telling me that the numbers looked great. The numbers continued to be quite high, pointing to a likelihood of twins (though the *experts* always claim that you can't infer anything from the numbers). But this was the only information we had to go on at this point until the first ultrasound which would happen at seven weeks, two days.

The week before the ultrasound, Dr. Zoumis' office called with the hormone results. The progesterone level looked great, but they had not yet received the beta hcg level because the lab had forgotten to run it "stat". The following Sunday, I saw Dr. Zoumis' number pop up on the caller ID. Thinking they must have finally gotten the beta hcg results, I rushed to answer the phone.

"Hi Honey, this is Grace from Dr. Zoumis' office." *Hi Honey?* The term of endearment set off alarm bells in my head. The person on the other end was clearly sympathizing with me because she was holding on to some really bad news. What now? Had the hormone levels fallen?

"Have you spoken to Tanisha?" Grace continued.

"No," I replied. Grace's question revealed more. I could see the angry bear resting on her tongue, poised to pounce on "Honey".

"Well, she called us last night because she was bleeding. It was more than just spotting, so we recommended that she go to the ER."

Grace's words bounced back and forth off the walls of my head, not knowing quite where to land. Having nothing to say, I waited for her to continue.

"At the ER, they performed an ultrasound. They saw two sacs, and only one had a heartbeat. They have done blood tests, but we don't have the results yet."

The ultrasound machine in my head played back the image of the twins inside of me, side by side, Ellie squirming and the other floating motionless. This image had been the first foreshadowing of the impending doom of the entire pregnancy. How could the same thing be happening in someone else's uterus? Was there just some rule that no child of ours would be allowed to enter the world no matter how safe a place we provided?

Grace assured me that they would call me with updates as soon as they heard any news. My paralyzed throat squeaked out a thank you. I hung up the phone, sitting motionless. It was bad enough that I had to give up my own dreams of pregnancy. The one silver lining of this whole thing, I had thought, was the high level of confidence in the outcome if the job were delegated to another uterus. We not only had the constant kick in the gut that our baby was not gestating inside of me, but now we also had the constant fear that the next heartbeat could be the last one. No matter what we did, the body count of our babies kept mounting. This put us at nine now. How long would it be before we had dead babies in the double digits?

When the day of the ultrasound appointment arrived, Tanisha's bleeding had stopped, and it looked like things were stable. But I knew that lack of bleeding was about as meaningful a predictor as a Magic Eight Ball. So many of my miscarriages never released a single drop of blood. As I arrived at the doctor's office, I stopped in the restroom. Staring in the mirror, I prepped myself for what I was about to see. I pictured both outcomes. A heartbeat would be a miniscule stepping stone in the direction of relief. But past experience told me that a heartbeat at seven weeks would only guarantee more worry the next time around. I turned and faced the darker possibility. What if we saw no heartbeat today? I told myself that I would try to view Tanisha miscarrying as a release from the moral obligation to use a surrogate. If we tried putting our babies in a woman with a proven track record, and she did no better than I did, then for the remaining embryos, we might as well just use me. This was a small positive that I could focus on to dull the pain of yet another child lost. Still aching to carry my own baby, it would be mildly comforting to view the failure of a surrogate as a license to put the remaining embryos in me. We would do every immune treatment possible to keep our babies alive. If that didn't work, then this struggle would be over once and for all.

So I gathered my courage and stood face to face with my ultrasound nemesis, prepared to survive whatever outcome it threw at me. Dr. Innis was very nice and seemed quite comfortable with surrogacy. This helped to offset my own discomfort. He quickly located the live fetus, and pointed out the healthy heartbeat. Smiling as he handed me the ultrasound picture, he said "Congratulations."

So that was that. I was granted a two-week reprieve until the next ultrasound. Two more weeks of thread-dangling hope. It did beat the alternative.

Chapter 41
A Year to Mourn

On November 5, I didn't realize that it was the one year anniversary of Ellie's death until I was in the car on my way to work. At that moment, the ghosts immediately flooded the car, drowning me in hazy shadow. They stayed with me throughout the day, and I cried off and on when no one was looking. Between weeping spells, I began to notice an urge building inside me. I felt like I should do something to mark the day, to honor my baby girl. But what could I do? She had no grave to visit. I didn't even have an image of her in my mind that I could visualize. I didn't want to talk about it with anyone because I didn't want to bring people's spirits down. They were most likely experiencing the day in blissful ignorance of its significance.

For some reason, a Filipino tradition came to mind. It is common in the Philippines for mourners to wear black for the entire first year after a loved one passes away. I had always thought that it was a bit of a morbid tradition that might trap people in a constant state of grief. I knew that I didn't have to wear black to remind myself to grieve for my baby. But on this day, I finally could see the wisdom behind the tradition. When the year was up, the black clothes would be put away, and color brought back to the world in a very tangible way. Maybe I could honor Ellie in that way, by somehow symbolically shedding the darkness of the past and bringing brightness back.

The idea came to me in a flash. I would let today pass and let the tears flow as they came. But tomorrow, I would initiate the first annual observance of Balloon Day. I would fill the house with colorful balloons and play with my family in the sea of color. After all, Ellie's life had ended on that day so that I would have a chance to remain alive and with our family. What better way to honor her sacrifice than to be completely present with my family? Upon seeing the colorful balloons and listening to my children's laughter, the black clothing of grief would make its way to the back of my closet. I would think of the joy that Ellie's brief life brought to our family. The bliss of her kicking inside of me. The thrill at my expanding belly. The milk that Ellie shared with her sister Natalie and might also share with the baby that was on the way. We would joyfully play together and celebrate our decision to let color dominate darkness. On every November 6 that followed, I would buy at least one balloon to remind me of my choice to honor my daughter by constantly focusing my life in the direction of brightness.

  So the next morning, I raced to the local party supply store after work and picked up two dozen balloons – 12 filled with helium and 12 that I would inflate myself. I came home, blew up the balloons, and hid the whole bunch of them in a couple of sheets (by chance, quite appropriately, the sheets which were available were decorated with images of the night sky). I finished just in time to pick the kids up from preschool. We went about the day, and luckily, the kids never ventured into my bedroom to discover the curious bundle. After James came home from work, I carried the huge mystery mass into the family room as the kids' watched with wide eyes. We counted to three, and I flung the night sky off, releasing the colorful swarm of balloons. Immediately, the room filled with shouts of glee and laughter, and balloons launched from every direction like an indoor fireworks display. The five of us played for hours. Marsha fell to the floor and hit the balloons up, keeping three at a time in the air. Jesse showed off his hitting and kicking abilities, as he and I worked together to keep his favorite blue balloon (which he named Anthony) from touching the floor. Natalie, being two years old, marched around collecting the helium balloons, informing everyone, "This is mine." James smiled and snapped pictures, launching any strays that came his way.

After a while, Jesse, the self-appointed Balloon Day Ambassador, began delivering helium balloons to various members of the family saying, "Happy Balloon Day." At that, Natalie started singing, "Happy Balloon Day to you…" complete with blowing out invisible candles at the end. This was my family, my reason for choosing life. I promised myself that as each new day presented its broad and unpredictable spectrum of colors, I would continue to choose life. No matter what.

Chapter 42
Recurring Nightmare

As the ultrasounds continued, so did the baby's heartbeat. Unfortunately, Tanisha's bleeding episodes continued as well, one of them severe enough to require an ambulance ride to the ER.

At the 14 week appointment, Dr. Innis noticed an abnormality while performing an ultrasound, and he referred Tanisha to radiology for a more thorough evaluation. Tanisha downplayed it when she described it to me, saying that it may have been some sort of leaking from the empty sac of the twin who did not make it. Lost twin, bleeding, abnormal ultrasound. I didn't need a time machine to visit the past. I was trapped in its endless loop.

As the technician performed the ultrasound, I dug each of my fingernails one by one into the thick crease of skin bordering my thumbnail. Despite my fidgeting fingers, I watched as though outside of my own body, removed from the ache that it was feeling. I slinked in the shadows and peeked at the beautiful baby on the screen who had perfect measurements, a vigorously beating heart, and Daddy's profile. An auspicious view between the legs revealed to my surprise that it was a boy this time.

Exploration into the abnormality was reserved for the final, tense moments of the ultrasound. As soon as the wand was focused on this area, I recognized the dark mass - the landscape of my recurring nightmare. There was no doubt in my mind. This was another hematoma. The technician took measurements and checked for blood flow as all had done before. I looked longingly at my son, who peacefully floated, unknowingly marked for the same fate as his sister. How could this be happening again? Was it possible that the problem wasn't actually my uterus, but instead was something inherent to the embryos created by James and me? Were our embryos somehow genetically poor at implantation no matter how fabulous of a womb housed them? This might mean that none of our jointly created embryos could ever survive. My gaze shifted to Tanisha. Was her life going to be at risk as mine had been? I couldn't take it if anything bad happened to her health due to this pregnancy. She had five children who needed her. What had we all gotten ourselves into?

As the technician withdrew the wand, I silently said goodbye to the son whom I had just seen, but would undoubtedly never meet. Dr. Innis called later and confirmed my diagnosis of hematoma, but he downplayed its severity, insisting that we just needed to keep an eye on it. He recommended another ultrasound in a couple of weeks back at the Stanford Prenatal Diagnostics Center, the same place that had monitored Ellie's hematoma. Couldn't the writers of my life story ever come up with anything new?

My daily life during this time period consisted of layers upon layers of stress. James and I were still mourning our previous seven lost pregnancies all the while anticipating the phone call that would announce the end of the eighth. At the same time, we were dealing with two special needs children, both with rigorous therapy schedules, both experiencing difficulty with self-regulation. As much as we adored Jesse and Natalie, it was very difficult to deal with the behaviors which went hand in hand with nervous systems badly damaged by meth-amphetamines. With two of them now to rile each other up, it was virtually impossible at times to get them to de-escalate.

I found myself less and less capable of keeping my cool as screams launched at me from every direction. At times, I would completely lose it and scream back at the top of my lungs. Looking into their fearful eyes, I would feel like the lowest form of scum on the planet. I marveled at my astonishing weakness of character. How could someone like me, who had waited so long for these precious children, turn around and take my own ineptitudes out on them? The thought would flash through my mind that this must be the reason that God was withholding a biological baby from me. I was such a poor excuse for a person that I must simply not deserve to have children. But at the same time, if I were so undeserving of a biological child, then why would God then go and entrust me with not one, but two special needs children? Further, if God were in the business of preventing bad people from becoming parents, then come on, there would be a lot more sterile people around. Then the thought would occur to me that maybe this wasn't so much of an effort to protect my progeny as it was to punish me for my sins – to hit me where it would hurt the most.

    At this point, I began to take some serious issue with the religious thinking that had been hard-wired into my brain from my Catholic upbringing. God was to be credited with and praised for all of the good things that happened in my life, and I was to be blamed for all of the bad. Whether this belief was correct or not seemed unimportant to me at this point. What I knew for sure was that it was not helpful to me in improving my shortcomings. The agitation that these beliefs generated was adding to the very frustration of which my children were taking the brunt. If I were to improve as a person and retain any sort of belief in a Higher Power, I would need to start viewing God differently. My current view cast Him as the polar opposite of the positive parent that I was trying to be to my children. I could not prevent bad things from happening to my children. Maybe God was also just an innocent bystander in the series of traumas that had taken over my life. I also knew that the best way to help my children to grow was to love them and encourage all of the good things they do rather than harping on their mistakes. Maybe I could do that for myself as well. Maybe I should just accept that I'm not perfect and instead of beating myself up over my weaknesses, just work hard to encourage my strengths. It was then that I decided that I would parent myself using positive discipline. Instead of delivering stern lectures to myself over bad parenting, I started rewarding myself for good parenting. I set up my own little rewards jar which I placed a quarter in for each day I was able to keep my cool with the kids. When the jar was full, I would treat myself to something. It wasn't that I really cared about the reward, but somehow just reframing my thoughts to encourage my improvements rather than reprimand my failures helped me to make some positive change. Of course I still had my bad days, but they were significantly diminished. I was steadily moving in the right direction.

Chapter 43
Closer

By the time the next ultrasound appointment rolled around, Tanisha had gone six full weeks without bleeding. That was a good sign, but I had learned not to read too much into signs. I fully expected to see my baby boy all scrunched up with inadequate fluid as Ellie had been at this point in my last pregnancy. However, to my surprise, the ultrasound revealed that the baby was still fine. The coloration of the hematoma indicated that it seemed to be resolving itself. An ultrasound four weeks later showed the hematoma had reduced in size. Six weeks later, the baby was still going strong, and the technician could no longer even find the hematoma. By this point, the pregnancy was 28 weeks along. Even if something were to go wrong, it would be safe to deliver the baby at this gestational age.

James and I dipped our toes tentatively in the belief that this pregnancy could actually be successful. We whispered the name Isaac once in a while. We were still constantly bracing ourselves for what would go wrong next. We were afraid to even make preparations for a new baby, but since the birth was now only 12 weeks away, we figured we better start thinking about it. So we finally mustered up the confidence to start organizing the rooms in the house so that he-whose-name-shall-not-be-uttered-aloud would have a place to be in the event that he actually showed up.

For the past year and a half, I had been pumping milk religiously for Natalie three times per day. I would pump once in the morning before work, once during the kids' nap, and once in the evening before bed. That was all I was willing to commit to long term. I brought the pump along on vacations, snuck off to the restroom during family gatherings, and hid under a blanket during long car rides. It had been a wonderful experience for Natalie and me. I loved being able to provide her with milk, and she heartily enjoyed the milk. Sometimes when she was sick, it was the only thing that she would be willing to consume.

Breast pumps are far less efficient than human babies. And although three times per day seemed like a huge commitment, my supply had gradually dwindled over time to just three ounces per day. I knew that I would need to ramp up considerably in order to be ready for a new baby, so when we hit the 30 week mark, I spoke with a lactation consultant. She recommended that I pump at least 100 minutes per day, and never let five hours go by without pumping. She felt that if I aimed for 19 ounces per day, I would have an ample supply for a new baby. So I rented a hospital-grade pump and began a rigorous pumping routine which included one 2:00 am pumping session per night. It was hard to keep this up and take care of the kids and home, but I figured I could manage anything if it was for only two months. As my eyelids got progressively droopier, I reassured myself that acclimating my body to nighttime waking at this stage would lessen the shock to my system when the baby came.

My milk supply increased at a frustratingly slow rate. By a few weeks into the effort, I had added every possible herbal supplement, then finally a medication called Domperidone to boost my supply. The Domperidone seemed to have the greatest effect. After only one week on Domperidone, I was pumping an additional three ounces per day, and my supply was climbing every day.

The conditioning of the past seven years had persistently reinforced the message that no matter how gentle the landscape seemed, James and I were always a few short steps away from a boiling lava pit. It was difficult to believe that we could ever have success when it came to reproduction. However, as the due date approached, I occasionally found myself entertaining thoughts which were founded upon the assumption that Isaac might actually survive as a nonvegetative human. This thinking brought up a set of new concerns.

One issue that required some thought was how we were going to inform people about this new baby. Up until this point, we had kept very quiet about what was happening. We had only told a handful of close family members and not until well after week 30. We hadn't wanted the burden of keeping a large set of people updated, especially when our sanity depended on being able to put the worries out of our minds. Most of all, we did not want a long list of people to inform in the likely event that the pregnancy failed.

What would we say to people if and when this new baby suddenly appeared in our lives? Did every neighbor, coworker, acquaintance, and remote family member need to know precisely how Isaac came to be? There was so much explanation required for a full understanding of our decision to pursue surrogacy. I knew that some people would never understand. For example, one of Tanisha's friends, upon hearing that she was a surrogate, responded with, "Don't you think that if God wanted them to have a child, He would have given them one?" *Ouch.* Even though I knew I could tunnel my way across the country with the holes in that logic, it still hurt to hear that. If God really were so powerfully involved in decisions of reproduction and so strongly wanted me childless, He could prevent my baby from surviving no matter who carried him. Also, if reproduction solely depended upon God's divine seal of approval, then theoretically even the smallest intervention to improve the odds of pregnancy, down to timed intercourse would be an attempt at undermining God's plan. I knew my close family and friends would support us. But the general population's convictions regarding surrogacy were unknown to me.

James and I decided that we had some right to privacy when it came to the general population. So we agreed that if Isaac did survive, we would announce his birth and allow people to draw their own conclusions about the steps leading up to it. Those who had not seen me in the past nine months might assume that we finally had a successful pregnancy, and those who had seen my non-pregnant belly might assume that we had done another adoption. If people chose to ask us, we would truthfully inform them about the surrogacy, but otherwise, we would leave it to their own vivid imaginations.

Another concern that had been bubbling up for a while was how Isaac was going to feel when he came into this world and had to separate from Tanisha and everything that was familiar to him. I wondered how we could make his transition into our family as smooth as possible. I remembered reading about studies in which brand new infants were able to clearly demonstrate recognition and preference to their birth mother and some of the familiar voices which they heard while in utero. My occasional lunches and ultrasound appointments with Tanisha would certainly not be enough to grant me residence in Isaac's auditory memory.

At some point, an idea began to take shape. James and I could make a recording of our voices. If Tanisha were willing to play the recording to her belly each night, we could possibly work our way into Isaac's inner circle of recognition. A quick online jaunt revealed that there were actually "belly headphones" in existence for this exact purpose.

The next question was what to record. If Tanisha were to play the recording to him each night, it would make sense to say goodnight to him in some way. The first thought that crossed my mind was to sing him a lullaby. Then after he was born, we could sing him the same song each night. I thought about the lullabies that were familiar to me, and none of them felt quite right. I didn't really find comfort in images of babies dangling precariously from tree-tops or descriptions of serially malfunctioning gifts such as mockingbirds and diamond rings. So I decided that I would write my own lullaby which expressed my nighttime wishes not just for Isaac, but for all of my children.

Over my lifetime, I had written a very meager number of songs. Typically I was unable to produce a song at will. I had to wait for inspiration to grab me by the collar when I least expected it and drag a song out of me. So I decided not to sit down and write immediately. I continued with my day, and a couple of hours later, as I was folding laundry, my mind started searching for images that might comfort a child who was about to go to bed. Immediately, one of my favorite children's books came to mind. *The Invisible String*, by Patrice Karst, describes love between people with the beautiful image of an invisible string which directly connects one heart to another. The string stretches with distance but never breaks the link between the two hearts. The image spoke strongly to me of my relationship with my children. Although we had never been connected through an umbilical cord, our love for each other still formed a permanent and powerful bond. As soon as I decided to respectfully borrow that image, the words to the lullaby came to me in one sudden flash:

> An invisible string, from your heart to mine,
> Throughout all of space, throughout all of time,
> Reaches over the mountains and under the deep,
> While you're awake and while you're asleep.
>
> So now as your lashes sweep down heavy eyes,
> Go run through the flowers and soar through the skies,
> And feel in the morning the sun's gentle touch.
> Oh beautiful baby, I love you so much.
> Oh beautiful baby, I love you so much.

I had no idea of the melody when I snuck away to our backyard music studio while the kids napped. But somehow, the moment my fingers made contact with the piano keys, the music flowed out easily as well. It was a simple song - exactly what I had been looking for.

James and I recorded the song over the next week. I hoped the sincerity of the wishes would make up for my weak and imprecise singing voice. Isaac would be stuck with me as his source of lullabies for better or worse.

Chapter 44
Lullaby Time

When Isaac's recording was complete and the belly headphones had arrived, I emailed Tanisha, hoping she would be willing to provide Isaac with his nightly uterine soundtrack over her last month of pregnancy. To my relief, she responded with her usual enthusiasm, saying it was a great idea.

Later that same day, I happened to run into Tanisha. I was speaking with a mutual friend when Tanisha walked by, shooting me a look of urgency. The friend greeted Tanisha with an unexpected question,

"Are they still six minutes apart?" the friend asked.

"Yep," Tanisha replied as she walked hastily past.

The friend turned to me, "She is not due for another month."

I practically swallowed my tongue as I took in the words I had just heard. My mind tried to grasp for some other explanation for this interchange besides the obvious. Struggling to maintain my composure with this person who was completely unaware of my deep connection to Tanisha, I responded, clasping my hands together to conceal the trembling.

"Oh wow," I said. "I hope everything goes OK."

I wrapped up the conversation with as much nonchalance as I could muster, and hurried off, whipping out my cell phone.

Tanisha answered with, "Hi, can I call you right back?"

"Um, Ok." I hung up, wondering if this kind of scenario is what causes the freak cases of spontaneous combustion that are reported from time to time.

Internal temperature rising, I called James. I could practically hear his pounding heart through the phone as I recounted the events of the past five minutes. Despite the struggle from each inhale to exhale, we hammered out a plan for the immediate future. James would sit tight at work, phone in hand, and I would pick up the kids, who were just about to get out of school. Next I would return home to hastily pack an overnight bag and try to secure a babysitter. That way, we would be somewhat prepared if we needed to rush to the hospital at a moment's notice.

As I drove, I attempted to process the jumble in my head. In a single moment, this seemingly ordinary day's potential had burst open in a wild explosion. What day was it anyway? Would this be his birthday? The excitement in my body lay in anxious wait like a runner on the starting line, aching for the release of the starting pistol. Would I be meeting my son before the day was over - seeing that precious face that I had spent the past seven years imagining? But reality rudely interrupted - it wasn't time yet. This wasn't supposed to happen for five more weeks! I knew that it would be relatively safe for him to be born at this point, but still not as safe as it would be in a few weeks.

After what seemed like an eternity, my cell phone finally rang. Tanisha sounded as calm as usual on the other end.

"I tried to come by earlier to talk with you, but I didn't want to alarm you right off the bat." *Too late – glass broken, alarm pulled.*

"I've been having some contractions, and I had a bit of spotting this morning, but I'm pretty sure they're Braxton Hicks. They are just not intense enough to be real. Still, I called the doctor just in case, and he wanted me to come by the hospital just as a precaution. I'm absolutely sure that they will send me home in a couple of hours, but I thought you should be prepared just in case."

OK mind, try to keep up. I felt like I had just been asked to perform a back flip midway through a front flip.

"Would you like me to come join you at the hospital?" I asked.

"No, that's not necessary." she replied, "Orlando is coming with me. We'll just hang out, and if anything changes, I'll give you a call."

I hung up the phone and tried to assess things. *This is good news. It is better if he waits until his due date.* But my heart slumped to the base of my chest as the image of the baby boy in my immediate future faded and blurred.

Still, I continued with preparations in case Tanisha's instincts about these contractions were wrong. I kept my cell phone in my jeans pocket as I gathered court documents, breast pumping supplies, important phone numbers, toothbrushes, and every other item that shot its way out of the brain chaos.

At 3:00, the phone rang again.

"Well, I guess you guys should come by the hospital," Tanisha said. "I'm three centimeters dilated, so they are going to admit me. Looks like today's the day!" *Are you freaken' serious?? This is it, this is it, this is it!!*

As James rushed home from work, the eager babysitting tag team consisting of my mom, my grandma, and my aunt assembled in my family room. When James arrived, we packed up the car, and soon we were driving. I slapped my face a couple times to make sure that this was not a dream. We were driving to the hospital to have a baby. James and me! Incredible!

At the hospital, we found Tanisha in a large labor room, hooked up to a fetal monitor and an IV. As usual, she was calm and cheerful, though a bit irritated at the hospital staff for not allowing her to get up and walk around. She complained that the labor may take all night if she weren't allowed let gravity do some work. Her husband and eldest daughter were both there, Ipods, magazines, and snacks close at hand, hunkered down for a long period of waiting. All of us sat together and had cheerful, friendly conversation. Each time a contraction would come, Tanisha would get quiet, as would the rest of us. Her face would tighten, and her body would freeze. The only sound in the room was the familiar scratching of the machine which recorded each contraction. As soon as it passed, Tanisha would calmly continue the conversation as though the pause button on the DVD had been released.

Each time a nurse or doctor came in to examine Tanisha, James and I would leave the room and retreat to the waiting room until Orlando came to fetch us. We appreciated the need to respect Tanisha's privacy, but the banishment accentuated the fact that we were the outsiders in this process, the last to know anything. Tanisha went to five centimeters dilation, then six. Things were moving faster than she had expected.

We returned to the room after one exam to find the tone had changed dramatically.

"I knew that they should have let me walk around," Tanisha ranted, "Why can't they just listen to me?"

"What's going on?" James asked.

"The baby is not head down any more." Tanisha pointed to her left hip. "His head is here, and his arm is down here. They want me to lie down in a different position to see if he will go back in place."

I regained my breath. That didn't sound too bad. Tanisha would turn to the side, and Isaac would float casually back into position. Not textbook perfect, but nothing to be alarmed about. Orlando stood next to Tanisha and calmly reassured her. We settled back into light conversation, and the mood of the room gradually improved.

The next time James and I were shuttled out of the room, we nervously waited for an update. We watched the door to the labor room. Different people moved in and out, but Orlando was never one of them. It became clearer that this situation was deviating further and further from the lines of the textbook. Why couldn't one single thing just go smoothly!

Eventually James and I stopped a nurse who was leaving Tanisha's room to plead for an update. To our relief, she was happy to fill us in.

"So the baby is not in the proper position. In order to deliver vaginally, he has to be head-down. What we are going to do is try to turn the baby and get him lined up properly. Tanisha has been given an epidural so that she will be relaxed and won't experience any pain while the doctors try to turn the baby."

"Is this safe for the baby?" James asked.

"The baby will be monitored closely throughout." She responded. "This is something that routinely happens, so the doctors have lots of experience doing this. If her water breaks or if there is any sign of fetal distress, then they will immediately move to a C-section."

"Wouldn't it be safer to just do a C-section now?" James asked.

"Well Tanisha prefers that we do all we can to make this a vaginal delivery." The nurse responded.

And of course, rightly so, the decisions were all Tanisha's to make because it was her body. Our preferences regarding our own child carried no weight whatsoever.

James and I sat silently in the waiting room, watching the door for any sign of Orlando. We waited. Like so many times in the past for an ultrasound, a test, a phone call. We braced ourselves, with only our past experiences to hint at the outcome. Was it possible that we had come this far only to lose another baby?

After what seemed like hours, but was probably more like 20 minutes, Orlando appeared at the door. For the first time, he appeared shaken.

"It didn't work guys." He said, "They are going to have to cut her open."

"Oh my gosh," my voice quivered, "Is she OK?"

Seeing the panic on our faces, Orlando quickly shed his own. "She's going to be fine. This same thing happened when my first wife delivered my daughter. It's a pretty common thing. You guys can come back to the labor room to wait with us."

As we walked, our son was somewhere in the building being delivered. He was somewhere close by, but it felt like light years away. We sat in the labor room with Orlando and Tanisha's daughter. The television was on, which prompted a discussion of politics. As we spoke, I marveled at how adept Orlando was at distracting us. Every once in a while, I checked my watch. A half an hour passed. Then forty-five minutes. How long was this supposed to take? I hadn't checked in a while when we were all startled by a woman entering the room. I searched her face for answers, but hers, like the faces of so many characters in our past, betrayed nothing.

"Mr. and Mrs. Aguas?" She said.

"Yes, that's us." I blurted as James and I scrambled to our feet.

"Come with me to the NICU." *The NICU!?!* Images flashed through my head of tiny, fragile babies under plastic cover and harsh lights, with tubes and wires and tape every which way. Was that how my son was going to look? What was wrong with him?

James and I hastily scooped up our things and followed the woman, who walked ahead, not looking back.

"Why is he in the NICU?" I could barely work the question out of my mouth.

No response.

The woman approached a door. As she opened it, she finally turned to us. A smile softened her stony face.

"Congratulations!" She said. *Ok, this feels a bit better.*

"Is he OK?" I stared at her, willing the answers out.

"Yes, he was just a little pale, so they admitted him to the NICU for observation."

My firm hold on my emotions gave way and my entire body began to tremble. Isaac was alive, and he was OK. And we were moments away from meeting him.

The woman instructed us to wash our hands thoroughly before entering the NICU. We held the hospital bracelets on our wrists up to the camera by the door, and a nurse from within activated the automatic door. As the door swung, I hastily scanned the room that it revealed. There were two rows of bassinets. Which one belonged to our son? A bassinet in the second row caught my attention. There were a couple of nurses attending to a baby as though he were the new kid on the block. But their bodies blocked my view of the baby. Our leader approached that bassinet, and as I walked, I craned my head from side to side to get a view of the object of all that attention. Finally, we reached the bassinet and got our first un-obscured view.

And there he was. He was lying on his back with a harsh light shining on his naked, scrawny body. His arms and legs flailed wildly. His entire body trembled. His face was contorted in a most unpleasant look of terror and frustration.

"You can touch him if you'd like." The nurse smiled.

James and I tentatively approached him and touched his soft, shivering body, trying to calm his panic. My hands were cold. I wasn't sure if I was comforting him or making things worse.

This is my son. I had to remind myself in order to believe this moment that my mind had walled off years ago as an impossibility. The baby in front of me was my son. Still, he felt foreign to me. In fact, how could I be sure this was really our child? I couldn't immediately see any resemblance to anyone on either side of the family. His wet, slightly wavy hair was honey colored, way lighter than I expected for a half-Filipino baby. His chin dramatically receded, lined with a deep upside-down U-shaped crease. There were large bags under the pained expression in his tightly shut eyes. I had to admit, this baby was kind of crazy-looking, like some sort of alien creature. I of course didn't care how my baby looked, as long as he was healthy. I just hoped that there was no mistake, and this was really our child. I warmed my hands on the lights above him, and continued to stroke his legs and feet.

A nurse working on Isaac looked up at our moist eyes and trembling extremities. "You've waited a long time for this little guy, haven't you?" She said.

James told a brief summary of our story as the nurses monitored Isaac and worked on his admission paperwork. He told them how we had been in that very hospital one year earlier with vastly different results. How we were bringing the milk intended for that baby to Isaac. Before he had even finished, Isaac's nurses were sniffling and blinking away tears.

Even the nurse attending to the neighboring baby made a quick retreat behind the privacy curtain. Our nurses teased him that he hadn't escaped quickly enough for his tears to go undetected.

At long last, a nurse uttered the words that I had been waiting to hear. "Are you ready to nurse him?"

Am I ever! Get that poor baby off of the unfriendly table and into my arms where he belongs!

The nurse skillfully swaddled him, put a knit cap on his head, and handed him to me. Now that he wasn't left to flail on the table, his face relaxed. No longer fighting against the bright lights, he even opened his little eyes a crack. I was shocked at what I saw as I looked into his tiny, almond-shaped eyes for the first time. It was James staring back at me, clear as day. In that moment, Isaac's looks suddenly made sense, despite the premature, old-man/alien-like features. I saw a bit of my father, a bit of my brother, but mostly, and very distinctly James. There was no mix-up. This precious, five pound bundle was undeniably ours. He could not have been more beautiful to me.

I jolted out of my reverie, remembering that the task at hand was to nurse this baby. I was eager, yet quite nervous that it wasn't going to work. I had learned by now not to blindly trust in the proper functioning of my body. Plus, I knew that preemies often had latching issues, and typically had to be bottle-supplemented. Early bottle feeding can cause babies to reject the breast altogether. Also, since Isaac had come so early, I was not anywhere near up to my goal of 19 ounces per day. I had worked so hard to keep my milk going and bring my supply up. I hoped that all that effort had not been wasted.

Awkwardly, I brought Isaac to my breast. The nurse, seeing right away that I had no clue what I was doing, gently took over. She repositioned my arms, bringing Isaac's head to my nipple. She moved his head back and forth and tried to entice him. Isaac slept away, paying no mind to our efforts. The nurse continued. Just when it seemed like nothing short of a drum and bugle corps marching through the room would interrupt his precious sleep, Isaac's primordial instincts suddenly kicked in, and he opened his mouth wide like an eager baby bird. He latched right on and started sucking with vigor, even swallowing one or two times. His baby gurgles and grunts delighted my ears. I braced myself for a lightning strike or a tornado. Could it be possible that the universe was going to allow me another victory in that same day? But the walls of the hospital stood firm while my son sucked up his first meal. He only lasted about 30 seconds before abruptly falling back to sleep, but it was arguably the most bliss-packed half minute of my life.

I was happy that Isaac was getting extra monitoring to ensure that he was healthy, but it was hard to leave him in the NICU. However, I couldn't stay in the NICU forever because I still needed to peek in on Tanisha and see how she was doing. When I entered her room, she groggily looked up at me and smiled. Careful not to jostle her too much, I hugged her.

"He is perfect," I told her between sniffles, "I don't know how to thank you for this. You have been so wonderful throughout everything. You are an absolute angel to our family."

Tears started rolling down Tanisha's cheeks. "He's a lucky little boy to be in your family. I'm so glad he's doing well." Her voice was weak and raspy, "I just wish I could see him."

Since Isaac was in the NICU, we unfortunately couldn't bring him out to see Tanisha. James had come by earlier and showed her some pictures of him, but she understandably wanted to see up close the child that she had carried for nearly eight months. The boy who would not be alive if it weren't for her. I assured her that we would bring him to her the moment he was released from the NICU, which would hopefully be soon.

I observed that she had a morphine pump hooked up to her. I hated to think of her being in pain. When I asked her how she was feeling, she said that she was doing OK. She said she felt more sore from the baby-turning efforts than she did from the C-section. Isaac also had bruising on his legs from the ordeal.

I could see that Tanisha was exhausted, so I didn't stay long. After ensuring she had everything she needed, I let her rest.

That night, I set an alarm to go off every two hours so that I could return to the NICU and nurse Isaac. If there is a heaven, then it must feel something like it felt that night sitting in that rocker with that baby, humming his first lullaby.

Chapter 45
Released

After two nights in the NICU, Isaac was thriving with no issues other than a touch of jaundice. At this point, he was finally released to the care of the regular baby nursery. As promised, we wheeled his bassinet straight to Tanisha's room. Her groggy eyes came to sudden attention as she caught sight of him.

"Aww he's beautiful guys!" she said outstretching her arms. I handed him to her, and he melted into her, continuing to sleep.

"Hi there little guy," she gently spoke, looking him over. She set him down on her abdomen and opened up his blanket.

"Oh, are you hurting?" she said as she stroked his bruised little legs. "I know just how you feel – we got roughed up by those doctors, didn't we?"

"I wish you would wake up so I could see your eyes," she pleaded with the doggedly sleepy boy. Clasping his hands, she softly sang happy birthday to him, gently moving his arms to the rhythm. Still no luck at cracking his determination to sleep.

I carefully watched her interacting with Isaac, wondering how it felt for her. As all of the post-partum hormones rushed through her body, did she feel like she was losing her own child? If she did feel any sadness, it was impossible to detect. Her face projected nothing but pure delight when she handed him back to us.

"Let me take a picture of the three of you," she said, reaching her arms out to our camera. The three of us huddled together, finally together, thanks to the beaming camera woman. It felt so good to sense Tanisha's happiness right there alongside ours. We were a team. We had stuck together through the rough battles, and it finally was time to bask in the most amazing possible victory.

After one additional day in the hospital, Isaac was cleared to go home. On that day, James and I made our first hospital exit accompanied by an actual baby. Since I was not a patient in the hospital, mine was not the traditional triumphant-mother-in-wheelchair exit that I had seen so many times. Instead, James and I walked out on our own steam, carrying the car seat containing our son. Our scene played out just as our life had - we could not sit back and ride the typical pregnancy and delivery experience as others could. We had to move mountains to make it happen.

Isaac came home to three welcoming older siblings. To my surprise, Jesse and Natalie didn't display any signs of jealousy. They were both thrilled to have a baby in the house. Jesse was particularly enthralled with his new brother, spending a good deal of his time staring at him and stroking his head. Natalie's affection was a shorter-attention-span version of Jesse's. She would snuggle next to him and say, "I love baby I-lak so much!" Less than ten seconds later, she would be off running around. Marsha was charmed by Isaac immediately. She appreciated the fact that he didn't scream constantly like the babies that she was used to around our house. He brought out the baby-lover in her who had been lying dormant, catching up with the kid-lover who had always been there.

Before Isaac's birth, I had spent a lot of energy worrying about the general public's response to the new baby's sudden appearance in our life. However, I was pleasantly surprised that our family, friends, coworkers, and acquaintances were pretty much universally thrilled for us. Those who learned of the surrogacy were overwhelmingly supportive. My fears of judgment and condemnation had been completely groundless.

We settled into our new life. Isaac was a very pleasant and easygoing baby. He slept well. He cried rarely. He was fortunate to be spared the agony of dealing with the drug exposure that his older siblings had gone through. It was a welcome change for us to be able to relax and enjoy his babyhood. We weren't frazzled and sleep deprived. We weren't afraid when the phone rang that someone would swoop down and take him away. James and I found ourselves double-checking our reality constantly. Our baby had made it into the world. Our family was happy. It just didn't seem possible.

I was never able to produce quite enough milk for Isaac, so from the sixth week on, I had to supplement with formula. But I continued to nurse him. Isaac and I both thoroughly enjoyed the experience, and he got a respectable portion of his milk from me. Ellie's gift to Isaac quickly transformed him into a healthy, pudgy little marshmallow man.

For so many years, I had wondered what it would be like to have a biological child. As I had expected, my love for Isaac was identical to what I felt for Marsha, Jesse, and Natalie. But the experience of finally seeing this little person who was a unique piece of James and me was intensely satisfying and downright fun. To my delight, family members' faces periodically popped out of Isaac's micro-expressions. The thought of how his personality would unfold, which traits and talents he would inherit from which loved-ones made me giddy with anticipation. I was even tickled when I discovered that Isaac had inherited a rather embarrassing trait from me in which his throat produces a funny clicking sound when he yawns. I wasn't glad he got that trait, but I can only describe it as a special connection.

By the same token, I have many special connections with my adopted children that I will never have with Isaac: The 400 square foot condo that I shared with Marsha when I was single and it was just us girls. Her support and love that never wavered as her parents wobbled and stumbled from one trauma to the next. The tiny baby under the blue blanket who saved us from completely losing faith in the world. The wide, Muppet smile that ended the long struggle to meet the precious girl whose very name brought back our belief in miracles. The intense bonding that was born out of the intense struggles that these three children experienced with us by their sides. All of these connections string together the diverse gathering of beautiful souls that we call our family. I wouldn't have it any other way.

I have put a lot of thought into what I have learned or gained from this experience. People say that struggles make you stronger. I think in some ways, I am stronger. I have proven to myself that I have the capacity to prevail after being beaten down in the most unimaginably brutal way. That does give me a certain sense of confidence. I think I also have gained some perspective as to what big problems versus small problems are, and I probably let the little things bother me less.

In other ways, I am weaker. I still feel pain during times when others feel great joy. My heart is missing the pieces where my children who have died once lived. I can't say that I'm better off from the experience. All I can say is that I'm still here and still experiencing.

For Mother's Day, a few months before Tanisha became pregnant, I had Jesse make cards for my mother and grandmother using watercolor paints. Naturally, he wanted to use all of the colors in the set to create his work of art. On my mom's card, he accomplished this. It turned out looking like an impressionistic smattering of every available color. It was actually quite lovely, and I could imagine art-lovers staring at it, pondering the deeper meaning. By the time he got to Grandma's card, however, he had managed to get all of the colors mixed together, and his painting looked like a giant brown blob. Luckily, brown happens to inexplicably be Grandma's favorite color because this painting was truly a work of art that only a grandmother could love.

On the inside of each card, Jesse dictated, and I wrote what he said verbatim. Both cards had similar messages. They were something to the effect of, "Happy Mothers' Day Grandma. Thank you. You're welcome. I love you so much. That's it. Love, J-E-S-S-E, that spell Jesse!" Pleased with

Jesse's creation, I set the two paintings out to dry. Looking at the two very different images, I began to think about my own life as a painting. All the colors had to be used in my painting – the bright ones and the dark ones. They were all a natural part of living in this world, a guarantee for all people. Some experiences would be bright and happy, but there would always be the dark streaks and spirals that would interrupt the experience of the pure light. I think my mistake had been similar to Jesse's mistake on the second painting – I mixed the colors up too much. Instead of simply experiencing the bright moments of pure joy, I would often let the dingy darks murk things up, leaving myself in a brown haze. In my dark moments, I tried too hard to force in the light and to see something bright being born out of the pain. But there are some experiences so dark that they simply cannot be seen as blessings in disguise, at least by the human-limited way in which I view the world. Searching for blessings that didn't exist never transformed my darkness into light. It just created a muddy and confusing mess, leaving me on a constant quest to right all of the wrongs, to force my suffering into something worthwhile. I have found that those shadowy experiences are best recognized and accepted as the darkness that they truly are. They are best left to float alongside the brightness, always present, but in their own separate space, not permitted to dim the rest of the painting. In that capacity, they do serve a purpose of contrasting with the light, so that it is more readily recognized and appreciated. However imperfect the product of my brushstrokes, the most important part is that I'm still here, with the people I love, painting away.

Apology and Epilogue

  I promised myself when I started this journey of writing that I would not offer a single word of advice. Weary of one-size-fits-all platitudes, I had set a goal to record my experience on paper and let those who endeavored to read it infer their own advice which fits for them. I apologize in advance, as I am going to break that promise for a few little morsels that I consider universal. Rest-assured, it will be brief...

To those of you who have a loved one suffering with infertility:

  Good luck. Infertile people come in all shapes and sizes. Some are nourished by fortune cookies. Others gag and vomit. Some of us need to talk about our experiences all the time. Others never. Some will talk, but only with specific people. Odds are, we won't tell you which we are or which you are. The best that you can do is let us know that you are present and give us the space to talk with you or not. And if we do, just know that as much as you may sympathize, you will never understand. There is no word or arrangement of words that can begin to capture the manner in which infertility infects our existence. But know that deep down, we appreciate your invitations to us, even if we do not accept them.

And to my dear Sisters:

  I am not going to pretend that there is any sort of wisdom that I can flick off of a magic wand to glitter-coat your nightmares. I will only leave you with two suggestions from my experience. First off, be easy on yourself. You are not the only person to feel poisoned by the triumphant glow of a *fertile belly. You are not the first person to have dark, ugly thoughts about strangers and loved ones whose only crime was to live happily uncursed. You are not evil or undeserving. These thoughts are way more common than you imagine they are. I have met scores of perfectly wonderful people who have had these exact thoughts. Be easy on yourself. Give yourself permission to skip the upcoming baby shower or baptism. If you need to steer clear of certain friends, family, coworkers, TV shows, or lunchroom conversations in order to take care of yourself, then do so without shame. Just try to put activities and interactions in their place that will sustain your spirit during this time.*

My second piece of advice is to believe. I'm not going suggest that you believe in the fairy tale moment just around the corner in which the jagged fragments suddenly rise from the darkness and stitch themselves together into a dazzling needlepoint reading "It was all for the best." If that happens, wow, good for you! For the rest of us, it really wasn't for the best. It sucked. But what I'm submitting that you can believe is that just as suffering will always exist, life also has an unending supply of happiness to offer. Happiness that can sit alongside the darkness, arm wrapped around its shoulder. Happiness so powerful that it can lure even the most obsessive focus away from the darkness in moments brief and sustained.

There, no more advice now, I swear.

As for me, my mission is mostly accomplished. I am quite proud of the motley bunch that James and I have laboriously assembled as our family. My daily life is filled with love, gratitude, and the experiences of motherhood that I treasure (of course, along with the occasional I-could-wring-their-little-necks moments). I would not trade the children I have for anything.

God and I have come to an agreement of sorts. This truce is only possible if I fend off all beliefs that attempt to explain suffering. For me, "why" questions and frustration are inoperably conjoined. My best experience of God happens when I turn off the thinking and simply let myself take in the wonder of the Divine. This practice is much easier said than done.

As far as I can tell now, I will face on a daily basis my grief for the children that are lost forever, for the untarnished experiences that I will never have. I still long to somehow bring my remaining embryos into the world safely. I still cling to the hope that someday, a miracle will occur and I will be able to bring my children to life through my own body. Pregnancy sightings still induce pain. But I have found that with a bit of practice, and a lot of patience, I can live peacefully side by side with these aching parts of me, with these holes.

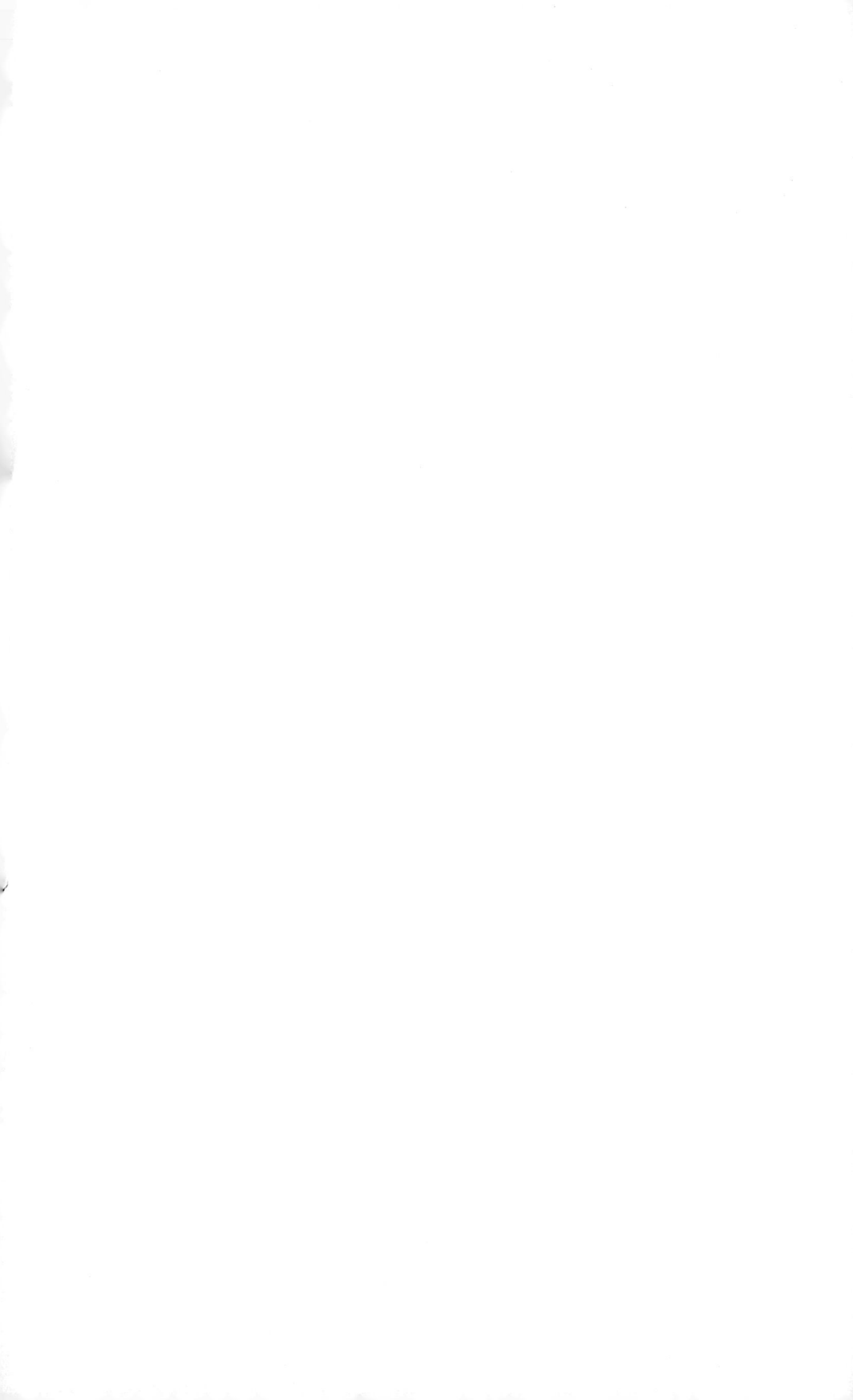

Made in the USA
San Bernardino, CA
07 January 2014